NEW YORK REVIEW BOOKS
CLASSICS

PROPER DOCTORING

DAVID MENDEL (1922–2007) was born in East London. He was a poor student and applied to medical school on a whim after discovering that he wasn't suited for his father's millinery business. He contracted tuberculosis while at his first hospital job and was confined to bed for six months, after which he spent time as a ship's doctor. In 1960 he was hired by St. Thomas's Hospital, London, where he would stay for more than two decades, working as a senior lecturer and a specialist in cardiology. During these years he wrote the well-regarded textbook *The Practice of Cardiac Catheterisation* and acquired a reputation as a popular and lively teacher. Mendel retired from medicine in 1986, moving to a cottage in Kent with his wife, Margaret, and earning a degree in Italian from the University of Kent. From then until his death he occupied himself playing the flute, building furniture, and publishing essays on Italian subjects, particularly about his friend, the chemist and writer Primo Levi.

JEROME GROOPMAN is the Dina and Raphael Recanati Professor at Harvard Medical School and chief of Experimental Medicine, Beth Israel Deaconess Medical Center in Boston. He has published more than 180 scientific articles, is a staff writer at *The New Yorker*, and most recently, the coauthor of *Your Medical Mind*.

PROPER DOCTORING
A Book for Patients and
Their Doctors

DAVID MENDEL

Introduction by
JEROME GROOPMAN

NEW YORK REVIEW BOOKS

New York

THIS IS A NEW YORK REVIEW BOOK
PUBLISHED BY THE NEW YORK REVIEW OF BOOKS
435 Hudson Street, New York, NY 10014
www.nyrb.com

Library of Congress Cataloging-in-Publication Data
 Proper doctoring : a book for patients and their doctors / by David Mendel ;
introduction by Jerome Groopman.
    p. ; cm. — (New York Review Books classics)
 Reprint. Originally published: Berlin : Springer-Verlag, 1984.
 Includes index.
 ISBN 978-1-59017-621-4 (pbk.)
 I. Title. II. Series: New York Review Books classics.
 [DNLM: 1. Physician–Patient Relations. W 62]
 R727.3
 616—dc23

                          2013015560

ISBN 978-1-59017-621-4
Available as an electronic book; ISBN 978-1-59017-643-6

Printed in the United States of America on acid-free paper.
10 9 8 7 6 5 4 3 2 1

CONTENTS

the Patient · Explanation · Reassurance · Helping the Patient
to Adjust to the Facts · If the Patient Rejects Your Advice ·
Drugs · Fatal Diseases and Death

INTRODUCTION

OVER THE course of their careers, physicians build a library. During the early years of medical school, they acquire foundational textbooks on anatomy and physiology, pharmacology and pathology. Later, in their clinical training, they add tomes on internal medicine, pediatrics, surgery, obstetrics and gynecology, neurology, and psychiatry. If they pursue a specialty, doctors complete their collection with volumes on that field, as I did in learning hematology and oncology.

Alas, another type of book often is missing from our shelves, a book like *Proper Doctoring*. In it, David Mendel, a British clinician, distills an oral tradition, passed down from eminent mentors, like in a guild, where masters offer unique insights to their apprentices. Such practical wisdom is as essential to the successful care of the ill as any formula about the contraction of the heart or knowledge about the behavior of blood cells in the bone marrow.

Proper Doctoring is written from the physician's point of view, and pulls back a curtain to reveal the delicate balance clinicians seek in their art. Mendel's overarching theme is medical professionalism, whose cornerstones are intellectual honesty and self-knowledge. He emphasizes that biases and preconceptions are at the root of misdiagnosis. Mendel further pinpoints the reasons that doctors may seek to be correct in their initial judgments, beyond the obvious benefit to their patients. He touches on the issue of physician ego as potentially interfering with sound thinking:

The only thing which pays dividends in the long run is getting the treatment right, and the way to do that is to get the diagnosis right, and the way to do that is to abandon your preconceptions as soon as you find they do not fit the facts. If you have made a terribly clever spot diagnosis you may be tempted to cling to it, bending the symptoms and physical signs a little to force them to fit, just for glory. But it is a mistake; proper doctoring demands total intellectual honesty. There is more than enough glory in getting it right.

Professionalism also dictates treating all patients with respect, and appreciating that the astute clinician can best uncover clues to a diagnosis by close listening to narratives. This is true even when patients express concern about the doctor's time being wasted with seemingly irrelevant talk.

Patients often apologise for wasting your time. Almost invariably it is the ones who are not wasting your time who apologise, and I always strenuously deny it...The patient has no way of knowing whether he is wasting your time or not, unless he is malingering and malingerers never apologise. Indeed, the longer they talk, the more certain the diagnosis becomes, so even then the time is often not wasted.

One of my mentors, Dr. Linda Lewis, a neurologist at Columbia University Medical Center in New York, told me: "There is nothing in medicine that is so complex that it can't be explained in understandable terms to every person. It's not rocket science." This places a burden on the doctor, because we become accustomed to communicating with colleagues using telegraphed jargon that is effective and efficient. But the people we care for typically lack this technical vocabulary. We then must formulate our phrases in a way that both sustains scientific accuracy and permits ready understanding. In essence, the physician becomes a translator who recasts patients' experiences in their own language. But there is an even deeper significance to my mentor's imperative. In order to explain a patient's condition in understandable terms, the doctor must have a deep familiarity with the biology of the problem and the rationale for the offered treatment.

Mendel echoes the injunction of Dr. Lewis, emphasizing that a medical professional must learn how to explain a malady, its cause and its course, as well as the rationale for its treatment, to anyone, regardless of background or culture. This accessible explanation by the physician should never be presented in condescending tones.

> Patients are drawn from the whole of the population, with its bell-shaped distribution of common-sense and intelligence. It is imperative to adjust your attitude and approach to each individual. This is not "talking down"—which is unacceptable, and which betrays dreadful intellectual snobbery.... A patient who is not as bright as you are may be your superior in every other respect. If the patient is a Nobel prize winner in physics, you still have to explain to him the nature of his disease and your reasons for advising the treatment.

Similarly, the profound uncertainty that pervades much of medicine should not be hidden from patients. This means that the words the doctor uses should specify what is known and what is not known, what is clear and what is intuitive.

> Our curious method of making decisions also determines what we say to the patient. As a lot of decision-making is based on guestimates, and other parts of it are the result of sensations which cannot quite be described, explanation is bound to be less than satisfactory.... Inadequate or incomprehensible explanations give no assurance. The explanation you give should aim at satisfying the patient, so that when you ask him if he has any questions, he says "No thank you Doctor, you have told me all I want to know."

My mother had an indolent form of multiple sclerosis that was initially misdiagnosed as "hysteria" when she became blind in one eye in her late twenties. Later in life, she was cared for by Dr. Lewis. After her appointments in the neurology clinic, my mother would call me and frequently remark, "I feel so much better after the visit." I asked what prescription she had been given, what new medication was administered. "No, Dr. Lewis didn't give me a pill. Just seeing her makes me feel better." Fortunately, my mother's case rarely necessitated active intervention; the risks of available therapies far outweighed any potential gains. One of Mendel's mentors was Dr. William Evans, and he cites him in a way that mirrors the words of my mother.

> William Evans used to teach that reassurance is the most precious pill which we administer. Many patients do not require any other medicine, but the "busy" practitioner often "saves time" by prescribing drugs which alter mood, in what he takes to be the appropriate direction. He then spends a great deal more time administering other drugs to counteract the side effects of the "mood benders," and the patient is no better for any of the medicines. When the patient can be satisfied with a verbal explanation, it is malpractice to administer drugs. William Evans coined the aphorism "It is better to do nothing than something, when nothing needs to be done."

Proper Doctoring also tackles the issue of conflicting information given to a patient. Mendel asserts the importance of designating a single physician to be in charge, who knows the patient well and can interpret divergent views. Still, second and even third opinions can be vital in deciphering an elusive diagnosis or presenting to a patient an alternative weighing of the benefits and risks of a treatment. Mendel, citing his revered mentor Dr. Geoffrey Evans, finds the cockiness that accompanies his good advice characteristic and amusing, but in doing so risks undermining how crucial the additional opinion can be:

Geoffrey Evans always welcomed a request for a second opinion, on the grounds that if the second opinion was any good, he was bound to confirm the Evans view, and that the consultation would serve as a subtle way of advertising just how good that view was.

Despite faltering here, Mendel quickly rights himself by explaining what kind of second opinion is most valuable.

A second opinion should be a good one and should be someone who the patient will find congenial. Whenever possible, he should be seen to be independent. Sometimes the patient will name the doctor he wants as a second opinion. In either case, the referring doctor is free to make it clear, in advance, if he disapproves of the second opinion, and he is free to accept or reject any new advice which may be given. If he rejects it, it should be rejected gracefully, and no pressure should be put on the patient.

Mendel terms "fringe" or "unorthodox" medicine what we currently label "alternative." He is appropriate in demanding that all forms of treatment must be scientific. But he also rightly goes further and affirms the value of an open mind.

One characteristic that all unorthodox forms of medicine have in common is that their claims to effectiveness have never been subjected to scientific evaluation. Enthusiasts for the methods, whether it be the suitability of whole foods for the whole man, or "nature's way" or the wisdom of the East, accept their chosen method for reasons which do not seem to be adequate to the impartial observer. Many of the claims do seem to be ridiculous, but some could be real. It is likely, for example, that a pharmacology based on Eastern plants will have some medicaments which are as potent as morphine but which Western physicians have failed to take up.

Doctors should know how they think, not only to avoid cognitive traps that can lead to misdiagnosis but also to maintain emotional equilibrium. We are typically driven students in the classroom and have rarely failed in the course of our studies. But over the course of a career in the clinic, failure is inescapable, and one of the most insightful observations from Mendel is how physicians may be tempted to displace their difficulty with admitting failure in a deleterious way.

> A doctor may find relief in telling the relatives that the patient is doomed, as a result of an incurable disease. This excuses the failure to cure which, in the present over-expectant atmosphere, may have made the doctor feel that his performance is not up to standard. Incurable diseases present a challenge to the doctor but he must beware of either "trying anything" to show that he has left no stone unturned, or unloading his feelings of failure onto the patient or his relatives.

Proper Doctoring is a book that should be read and then reread, first early in medical school, then later in clinical training, and once again as a seasoned physician. Laymen will also benefit from its acute insights, as it offers a window into the complex and uncertain world of care, where men and women in white coats strive to alleviate suffering and restore health.

—JEROME GROOPMAN

PREFACE TO THE
2013 EDITION

I MET David Mendel in 1976 near the end of his highly successful career in cardiology. He told me then he had "done" cardiology, as indeed he had. After a sabbatical at Oxford University, David then became the first person in the U.K. to record the surface potentials of the auditory system, the auditory brainstem response (ABR). Odd for a cardiologist to want to do this perhaps, but David's lateral thinking led him to this goal, in case he could use it as a model of neural function to test cardiac drugs. It wasn't useful for this, but it began his second career in auditory neurophysiology, and ensured that we became firm friends, and he my mentor. He learned the technique of ABR from Haim Sohmer in Israel, the first in the world to achieve it. The trick was the need to prepare the skin really well before applying the electrodes; advice ignored by others!

Although David kick-started the ABR in the U.K., soon to be used for measuring hearing impairment in premature and newborn babies, his real contribution to medicine was his great humanity and understanding of what it was like to be ill. As a young doctor, like some of his colleagues, he had spent a year recovering from tuberculosis. He had some truly great and inspiring teachers whose advice is repeated often in this book.

We spent many pleasant hours together in his lab at St. Thomas's Hospital; at his beautiful cottage in Kent, greatly enhanced by his own skills in joinery; and on conferences abroad mostly concerned with electrophysiology. A constant topic of conversation was the philosophy of medical practice. A constant delight was the presence of his wife, Meg, the ultimate hostess.

It was during a trip to Italy that David became irritated by his inability to speak fluent Italian. During a post-congress tour of the Palladian villas near Venice he decided something had to be done. On retirement he enrolled as an undergraduate at Kent University and attained a very creditable degree in Italian. His command of the language was further refined by frequent visits to Italy. He became a world authority on the works of Primo Levi, whom he greatly admired and who became a personal friend. He did not believe that Levi's death was a suicide and put up a very good argument to prove his belief. David became a skilled and much sought after broadcaster on the BBC.

I am delighted that this wonderful book, which I helped to persuade him to write, is being published for a second time. Although some of the techniques and treatments described belong to an era now past, the message of how to be a "proper," humane doctor is more important today than it ever was. The lure of technological advances in medicine and surgery, together with the economic constraints placed on everyone in health care, make it all the more important to remember the patient. If you follow the wisdom in this beautifully written book, you too can become a first-class doctor.

—Jonathan Hazell, FRCS

PROPER DOCTORING

To Geoffrey Evans, my teacher

"People come to us for help. They come for health and strength ...
There is an emotional or nervous aspect to all disease. We doctors
must be able to treat this. The basic weaknesses of human nature are
fear, self-pity and self-indulgence. Tennyson wrote in 'Denone':

Self-reverence, self-knowledge, self-control,
These three alone lead life to sovereign power

As medical students you can already contribute to your patients' re-
covery on this super-sensuous level. You will contribute to their self-
reverence by treating them with respect and understanding, and by
giving them their due in admiration for such fortitude (for instance)
as they show in suffering. You will be able to give them self-knowledge
by giving them such simple information on physiological principles
as is well within your knowledge and directly applicable to their sensations. You can give them self-control simply by having yourselves
under perfect control, control so perfect that you are not (for instance) irritated by an irritating remark. If a man has no money,
he cannot give it away. It is the same with these super-sensuous
things ..."

*(From a leaflet for students written by Geoffrey Evans
in the nineteen-thirties)*

PREFACE

THERE are many textbooks which give detailed descriptions of the causes, clinical features and treatment of disease. There are a number of books devoted to clinical methodology which tell the student the questions which he must ask and describe the physical signs that he should seek. The authors of these books rarely devote more than a page or two to a job description and advice on how to acquire clinical skills. Although a sound knowledge of the facts is essential, a good doctor differs from a bad doctor more by his attitude and craftsmanship than by his knowledge. These important matters receive scant attention in the textbooks because the authors regard them as part of the spoken tradition which is taught at the bedside or in the clinics and is absorbed by watching clinicians while they are dealing with patients.

The image of the doctor who greets patients with his pen poised over a prescription pad, and the calls for holistic medicine, imply that a number of students do not pick up the relevant attitudes and skills on the way. That this feeling is shared by the profession itself is suggested by the formation of a society to promote the treatment of the whole patient, and another for the promotion of humanism in cardiology. Good doctors have been treating the whole patient humanely since the profession was founded, and I find it shocking that it is thought that such societies are necessary.

Many of the attributes which make or mar a doctor are acquired before he reaches medical school, but they can be changed by training. Certainly techniques can be learned, and this book is an attempt to clarify and modify the reader's attitudes to what he does, so that he can turn knowledge into effective treatment.

The book consists of "points" which I learned from my teachers or from experience and are included because I feel that they will be useful, and are not usually found in textbooks. The length of each section is related only to the number of points to be mentioned and the number of words which it takes to make them. The fact that only twenty lines are spent on Past History means only that I have little to add on that subject to what is found in the textbooks; the brevity is no measure of the importance I attach to it.

It has not escaped my notice that approximately half of the patients and half of the readers of this book are women. When I started to write it I found that constant repetitions of "him or her" seemed obsessive. I then tried to alternate references to the sexes, but in the end I decided that this was a more sexist approach than to refer to everyone as "him."

—DAVID MENDEL
London 1984

ACKNOWLEDGEMENTS

THIS BOOK owes very little to the written word. The opinions found in it are my own, and I learned many of them from my teachers by word of mouth. Often I have modified what I was taught or extended it. In the course of a career one picks up many tips, and it is difficult to be certain of the origin of each one. The teacher who had the most profound effect on me was Geoffrey Evans. His views on the doctor–patient relationship and on history-taking were my guide. The things he said about physical examination have not had as much effect on me as did the teachings of Paul Wood, who most influenced me in that field. Neither of them left a lasting impression on my views about treatment; not treatment in particular, but advice and treatment for patients in general. Here my main influence was William Evans. I had not realised this division until I came to write the book, and found that the majority of references to each teacher was in different sections. Malcolm McIlroy influenced my attitude to test and Wallace Brigden is another man whose teaching has influenced my attitudes. There are many others, both teachers and colleagues, who have influenced me, and I am deeply grateful to them all.

Like most books which are manuals rather than treatises, the book contains no references. As I have said, it is based on the spoken rather than the written tradition and although there are studies on these matters, it did not seem worth citing "evidence" that patients prefer it if you are nice to them or if your stethoscope is warm.

A number of friends have been very generous with criticism and suggestions for the book. Foremost among these is Mike Matthews, who really should have been coauthor. He made innumerable suggestions and criticisms which I have tried to meet. Ivor Gabe, Alan Grimes, Zarrina Kurtz, John Lipscombe, Charles Nicol and John Scopes have helped me greatly. I am indebted to Jonathan Hazel, with whom I often discussed my views and who suggested that I write them down.

Finally I am grateful to Jane Farrell of Springer's editorial staff for helpful suggestions, and to Mrs. Barbara Issom who typed the manuscript.

1. THE JOB DESCRIPTION

THE PRACTICE of medicine is one of the most rewarding jobs in the world. The subject is fascinating, and it gets more interesting every year. The patients are all different and so are their diseases. Diagnosis and treatment are a challenge to the mind and, in addition, a job well done is rewarding on all levels: you have done well, the patient thinks you are marvellous and you think there might be a grain of truth in his opinion, you have done a bit of good, you have struck a blow against disease, and you may have shown your colleagues a clean pair of heels in the process. Curiously, one is well paid for all this enjoyment. Surely the boring jobs should be the best paid.

One absolutely essential ingredient of proper doctoring is the much-maligned bedside manner. The best doctors acquire one over the years, but many never do. I think that this is due to the usual overswing of the pendulum. Around the turn of the century, medical remedies were not very effective; in the circumstances the bedside manner was all there was. Now that we can cure many diseases, both doctors and public have replaced the wise avuncular physician of the past with the "intensive care whizz-kid" image. We don't need all that mumbo-jumbo when we have proper scientific methods, they say. Bedside manners, along with other manners, are at a discount. From the mechanistic viewpoint man is seen to be much like a motor car: you do a few tests, make the diagnosis, apply the appropriate treatment and all will be well. Nothing could be further from the truth; the mechanistic approach is usually insufficient, and it requires the addition of an effective bedside manner to make it work.

Science has made, and will continue to make, a fundamental

contribution to our understanding of disease. It is one leg of the medical couch. But reliance on scientific medicine alone is like lying on a one-legged couch. The other three legs are wisdom, experience and caring. For proper doctoring you need all four. At all stages in the doctor–patient relationship, from the initial interview to the patient's discharge, countless minor points of a non-scientific nature summate to produce good patient "handling," and that handling is in many cases as important as selecting the right drug; indeed, you may learn something which actually helps you to determine which is the right drug. The whole aim of proper patient handling is to maximise the effect of treatment. It's more efficient and, dare one say it, more human too.

THE IMPORTANCE OF COMMON-SENSE

Good doctoring is based on common-sense (which is much the same as judgement), intellectual honesty, self-discipline, sensitivity, enthusiasm, compassion, care, memory, reasonable intelligence and training. Medicine is not a very intellectual subject; most of the concepts are simple. Laymen and many doctors think of medicine as being largely a question of knowing enormous numbers of facts, and fitting them together like pieces of a jigsaw puzzle. There *are* enormous numbers of facts, most of which we do not yet know, and many of those we think we know are wrong, but the good doctor works with a tidal air of information which bears little relation to the vital capacity. Of course a good memory, particularly of patients, is invaluable, but failure of judgement is a more common cause of error than lack of information. None of these requirements is in any way exceptional. No "gifts" are required and this puts the job within the range of the well-motivated average student.

Common-sense, that most uncommon virtue, is the main ingredient, and because it seems so ordinary, it is not stressed enough. In medical training the accent is on facts, especially in the pre-clinical years, so the student gets out of the habit of using his common-sense. Like almost every other skill, common-sense is partly a matter of inheritance and partly of practice. If you don't use your common-sense it atrophies. If you do, and you are averagely gifted, you can work it up into a very adequate instrument.

Although many of the techniques necessary for proper doctoring are simple common-sense, many of them would not come to mind because they are outside one's experience. Most of us are not very good at putting ourselves in other people's shoes, and hence we have to be told what is really only common-sense. The doctor who contracts a disease himself gets a flood of new insights into a condition which he has been treating for years. It is a pity that getting all the diseases cannot be made part of the medical training. The curriculum is grossly overfilled, and teachers often, entirely reasonably, take the view that in the short time available it is more important to teach the students that oxygen therapy may lead to coma and death in the emphysematous than it is to teach medical good manners which are "only common-sense anyway" and which the student "will pick up on the way." Many students, pointed by their teachers along this mechanistic road, never learn how to handle patients properly, and their performance and their patients suffer.

POLISHING YOUR PERFORMANCE

The rewards of medicine only come from doing the job as well as you possibly can. Less than top performance is not only unrewarding, it is depressing. With each patient you have dozens of opportunities for doing well, or not so well. As in golf, each stroke counts and you don't get a chance to play it again. If you want to get round in par for the course, you cannot afford to muff a single shot. Whatever level you are at now, enthusiasm and relentless pursuit of excellence will reduce your handicap. Medicine is to be practised like a favourite game. Each patient presents another opportunity for a *tour de maître*. Seize it with both hands. Aim to go on polishing your performance until you retire; your self-respect demands it. At the age of eighty, Pablo Casals was found by an admirer practising slow scales. When the visitor expressed surprise, the cellist said "I practise the cello as though I am going to live for 300 years." And in cello playing nobody's life is at risk.

CRAFTSMANSHIP

Craftsmanship has overtones of ill-made goods bought in tourist shops, which fall to pieces when you get them home. These amateur productions belie the word craftsmanship, which applies to skilled work faultlessly done. I asked a silversmith if it would be "right" to fill in with silver solder a hairline crack inadvertently produced while making a silver teapot. If the teapot was then silver-plated, no one would be the wiser. As the silver solder contains a tiny amount of adulterant, the hairline crack would not be solid silver. The amount of adulterant in a hairline crack would, however, make no material difference to the total amount of silver, but I wondered whether he felt that morally one should scrap it and start again. He asked me why anyone should make a crack in the first place, and no matter how hard he tried he could not bring himself to imagine a situation in which he would make a crack, and hence he had no idea what would be the correct moral response if one did make one.

The essence of craftsmanship is to do the job properly. Producing a crack is botching the job, and craftsmen don't do that sort of thing. Many of the techniques in patient handling are craftsman skills. Of course the job is more difficult than silversmithing, but if you take a craftsman's pride in servicing the patients, you can keep the number of hairline cracks to a minimum.

PATIENT HANDLING, OR WHY MEDICINE IS NOT MECHANICS

If something is wrong with your car and you take it to six different, honest and efficient garages, the diagnosis will be evident from the symptoms and signs; the remedy advised at each garage will be the same, and the cost will be reasonable; if not, you abandon the car, without too much regret, and buy another. I admit that almost every clause in this last sentence is only partially true, and as Richard Asher said in his book *Talking Sense*, the motor car analogy is not a good one for human disease. Asher said that the analogy is true only in that in difficult cases both frequently had to be sent back to their maker. But I want to pretend for a moment that the sentence is entirely true, because it sums up the special difficulties of doctoring.

In medicine, in sharp contrast to motor repairs, many diagnoses are uncertain, and the agreement between clinical and post-mortem diagnoses is mortifyingly small. Medical knowledge is extremely uneven. Sometimes we understand almost everything about a condition and we may know how to cure it. For other conditions our knowledge is incomplete or fragmentary, and much of the evidence appears to be contradictory. In general, it is likely that our ignorance will prove to be much deeper than our knowledge. This makes the doctor's job very much more difficult than that of a garage mechanic, who can usually arrive at a correct diagnosis on a basis of almost complete understanding of how a car functions. Secondly, the treatments advised may vary greatly. Thirdly, the cost to the patient in terms of pain or unpleasantness or anguish may be considerable. And finally, you cannot send the incurable patient to the breaker's yard.

For these reasons, and because patients are not inanimate objects like motor cars, a sound knowledge of history-taking, physical signs, differential diagnosis and treatment, even though it is combined with infinite good-will, a saintly nature and common-sense—a rare combination indeed—is not enough to get the job done properly.

The techniques of dealing with patients have to be learned if the patient is to be made as well and as happy as the disease and the best medical treatment will allow.

As everyone is different, and as everyone's disease is different—a fact not yet fully known to the head-counters and drug-triallists—no book can give a magic guide to everybody, but there are a number of basic techniques which will give you a foundation on which to build your own practice. You will have to make modifications to suit your own personality and the needs of each individual patient. If you are gifted with great insight, and nine people out of ten feel that they have more insight than the norm, you will not derive much benefit from this book. Learning to be a proper doctor is analogous to learning to play a musical instrument: the really gifted seem to pick it up without tuition, but most of us require lessons. With the right motivation most of us in the end get to an acceptable level of competence; some get to be virtuosi and that is the level to aim at.

THE DOCTOR–PATIENT RELATIONSHIP FROM THE DOCTOR'S END

The relationship between a doctor and his patient is an extraordinary one. It is a voluntary contract based on a different set of rules from those which govern relationships between master and servant, shopkeeper and customer or man and wife. Being a doctor is not as demanding as being a fireman or a lifeboatman, who risks his life for strangers, but it is not like selling soap. Even the relationship between a lawyer and his client is limited to intellectual and emotional commitment. The doctor–patient relationship is based on the principle that the patient needs help, and that when called upon, the doctor will leave no stone unturned to make sure that the patient gets all the help that medical science can provide, almost regardless of expense. The patient expects this, and the doctor, if he is any good, has only to be approached, by a complete stranger, before he unleashes this flood of aid (generally paid for by the state or by insurance companies) for the benefit of "his" patient. It is extraordinary how any patient becomes "my patient," to be helped to the hilt, as soon as he steps into the consulting room. And in the best hands, this is true even when doctor and patient do not actually like each other.

There is no other situation where this beneficent relationship between perfect strangers comes about. Of course people will do much for someone they love, or for profit, or for their beliefs, and a small percentage of very highly principled people will devote their energies and their lives to some form of doing good, but these are exceptional people, and one does not *expect* that level of performance—one is simply amazed and delighted and humbled when one meets it. The great majority of doctors are not that exceptional but the great majority of people expect them to act in this unusually "involved" and "public-spirited" way.

A good doctor responds to the patient's needs in spite of the fact that life around him seems to be based on totally different principles, which each year seem to become more selfish and inconsiderate. Having put up with the careless or rude or hostile attitudes of fellow commuters, public transport personnel and shop assistants, one arrives in Outpatients and somehow contrives to act in a doctorly manner. As the climate of unashamed self-interest mounts, it must be more difficult for new generations of students to act up to the doctor's role than it was for earlier generations who were brought up to believe in duty and service, and that privilege involved responsibility. Whether they acted according to these increasingly unfashionable concepts or not, the feeling that they should be doing so set a standard much nearer to that which is still required from the doctor's end of the relationship. The patient's end too has changed in the same ways, and the modern patient with his often unfulfillable expectations and his "right" to perfect health, makes the doctor's role even more difficult.

DOCTORS AND THE MEDIA

In the last twenty years or so there has been a deterioration in the "press" which doctors have been getting. This does not by any means indicate that patients have lost faith in their doctors or necessarily that standards have dropped—though I believe they have—but in the media, and on social occasions, one constantly faces "knocking" references to all sorts of doctors. Much of the knocking has to be discounted. It is in the spirit of the times to knock the establishment of which doctors are seen to be a part. It is also in the spirit of the times to question authority even if you have no relevant questions, and if only to show that you are not the sort of muggins over whose eyes the wool can be pulled; knocking everything has become a way of life. As in so many spheres, in medicine the knocking is self-destructive because the one thing the patient really needs as recipient of our well-intentioned, but often sadly half-baked advice, is confidence in his doctor.

Fortunately, mother nature, in her infinite wisdom, does seem to affect people's minds when they become sick, and with commendably enlightened self-interest the sick patient very often abandons a lifetime of knocking the doc and assumes a faith in his own particular doctor which often surpasses understanding. One is forever meeting people socially who have just been treated who say "Of course you know Dr. (or more often, Mr.) so-and-so," whom they regard as the best in the country. They look disappointed if you have not heard of him (mostly one has not heard of him even when he is said to be in one's own speciality), and it is important to bolster the patient's faith in his doctor, so I say that although I don't know him personally, he is one of the leaders of the profession. The patient has a vested interest in being under the best man there is; it would be foolish of him in such a matter of life and death to go to anyone less good, so he promotes his doctor to "Top of the Docs."

TOO CLEVER BY HALF

A lot of gifts, like beauty or skill at games or academic brilliance or even being born rich, have distorting effects on the mind. The possessors of such gifts are led to believe that they are exceptional—as indeed they are—and they are often feted and flattered because of it. The gift may become their main preoccupation. The talented young often have high expectations, the "brightest chap we've ever had here, should go far" syndrome. And if they don't go far, and they often don't, because talent is not the main determinant of distance travelled, there is a sense of failure or of some injustice.

Sometimes a gifted person with insight comes to realise that his talent is not all that important and may feel unable to live up to his reputation. This may make him withdraw and appear aloof; the less you say, the less you reveal.

The gifted often exude an aura of success and self-sufficiency which cuts them off from ordinary people. This aura makes people feel that their usual conversation simply will not do and in striving to find something brilliant to say, they become tongue-tied. The gifted may become addicted to applause and do almost anything to satisfy the craving. In medicine, where common things commonly occur, they make fanciful diagnoses to impress the patient or their colleagues. A less gifted physician will get more satisfaction from getting the diagnosis right. If the gifted are narcissistic they use everything as a mirror to show themselves off to best advantage. They see patients primarily as reflecting surfaces, and this prevents them from looking inside and understanding.

The talented may feel that other people are cast in the role of acolytes, and that although admirers naturally want to know how their hero ticks, the fans are not interesting enough for that feeling to be reciprocated. The gifted doctor may share the view that the way he ticks is really rather absorbing and this widely shared interest in himself may prevent him from looking outwards, or having curiosity about others. What patients want of a doctor is concern with their own affairs. You have to listen to them and actually be interested in what they are saying, and actually want to know what they think and what is troubling them, and you have to care whether or not they are satisfied with the service that they are getting from you. This sort of mutuality is impossible if you have previously been led to believe that you are the star and that their job is to admire.

We all start off thinking that we are the centre of the universe and one of the great advantages of not having any talent is that you are forced to realise your insignificance at an early age. This makes for a speedier and more comfortable journey from the centre of the universe to the realisation that you are just a blade of grass. A proper doctor does not feel himself to be special but finds life special and people and their goings-on the most special thing of all. If this broad-mindedness is combined with what horsemen call in their mounts "good temperament," then it is likely that the possessor of these psychological gifts will turn out to be a proper human person.

One of the most useful realisations in life is the relationship between effort and achievement; a gift is almost by definition effortless and as effort is anyway tiring and often boring, the ungifted are often discouraged from trying. It would of course be lovely to have some or even many executive talents, but there is always the danger that the silver spoon will stick in your throat.

THE NEED FOR ROLE-PLAYING IN MEDICINE

Egalitarians believe that the caste system is based on false values, and in attempting to introduce more truthful relationships they condemn the element of charade in role-playing. Whilst hypocrisy is odious, it is absurd to go to the other extreme. Role-playing, with its inevitable less-than-complete truthfulness, is an integral part of the art of medicine.

The immensity of the decisions that a doctor must make and which his patient must bear, plus the fact that life itself may—though not as often as we like to think—depend on the decisions taken, mean that the doctor cannot play his role in the same way that the skilled mechanic can. Motor cars have no feelings, they have no opinions; and their ills are almost completely understood. So the successful doctor—and by that I mean the one who is successful in doing as much for his patients as medicine and the state of the latter's health will allow—cannot sail in on a call-a-spade-a-spade, cards-on-the-table basis.

Doctors vary in the extent to which they act. Some ham it up. Others are to the manner born, and practise their art without artifice. Some confine their role-playing to their work; others never stop acting. Doctors range from the saintly and perceptive who do not need to play-act, through to the horrid and insensitive, who may neither realise, nor care, how beneficial a role could be.

Taken overall, doctors are at least as nice as patients. Very few misanthropes or sadists take the job on, and not a few enrol to do a bit of good. Nevertheless, a doctor may not like a patient: he may be prejudiced against, say, Christians or white men; the patient's behaviour may be inexcusably offensive, demonstrating a curious lack of self-interest. A doctor's day may have started badly—arriving in Outpatients bad-tempered, cold and an hour late as a result of a row with his wife and a rail strike, he may not feel enough loving kindness to act as a buddy.

The answer is to have a bedside manner that is donned with the white coat. When my old hero, Dr. Geoffrey Evans, qualified, he examined his personality, found it unsuitable for healing the sick and changed it. He adopted a new role because he believed that the doctor's job is to make the patient as well and happy as nature and medical knowledge allow. This involves a never-ending study of patients' reactions, requirements, fears and feelings and of every aspect of one's own performance.

If you are unwilling or unable to play a role, you can improve your performance if you regard methods of handling patients as techniques. Some low-intensity early diastolic murmurs are inaudible unless you make the patient sit up and breathe out. You will not be able to hear them unless you adopt this technique. Similarly some patients will not tell you about symptoms which embarrass them unless you appear to be unhurried and sympathetic, and if you want to hear about these symptoms, you are forced to behave in a manner which will allow them to be revealed.

Nothing is worse than bad role-playing, because it is obviously phoney. The long years of training allow you to perfect your role gradually, and with increasing experience you take on more difficult roles. No one asks a student to explain to a patient that he is to have a leg amputated, but there is room for less demanding role-playing from the first contact with patients.

REHEARSING YOUR ROLE

The role of doctor, like the role of Hamlet, is not one which you can leap onto the stage and perform. In order to play Hamlet, as distinct from watching him which anyone can do, you have to examine each word, each phrase, and take it all in the context of the whole play. Each word, each tone of voice, each pause has to be *performed* in order to put over what the Bard had in mind. If you or I did it, it would produce a thoroughly boring evening in the theatre, but a professional, or better a great professional, makes it electrifying even if you have seen it nine times before. A great performer becomes great by talent and practice. Almost all great performers, and almost all professionals too, remain on top form by relentless attention to detail. If you watch musical master-classes you can see that the teacher seems to be entirely devoted to interpreting the work as the composer wished. He has an overall strategy and, as tactics, he considers how each individual note should be played. It is this remorseless attention to detail, before the actual performance, which makes a great performance.

Similarly in medicine, treating patients starts long before you set eyes on them and begins with a lot of training, but above all with a professional attitude towards the patient. However distinguished you are, the patient is the star and your role is to serve him. You will leave no stone unturned, from the moment he steps into the consulting room, to do your best for him, as if he were your nearest and dearest. And your best means playing every note right, with the right emphasis, tone-colour and touch, not only on the first visit, but on each subsequent visit—and you may treat him for twenty years or more.

It is impossible to do these things unless you make two major adjustments. The first is to change from one's normal self-indulgent attitude to a self-disciplined one. This term is not a popular one at present, and there are many occasions when self-discipline is not too important, but in medicine it is essential. Failure to cure a patient frequently occurs, simply because many conditions are incurable, and a doctor, though saddened at such a failure, need not feel as though he has failed personally. But a failure in professionalism, even if it results in a cure, should haunt a doctor forever. It happens to most of us, but it happens less often to the more professional, and one must aim at never letting it happen at all.

So you go on stage, knowing your role, knowing what you want to achieve—the perfectly treated patient—and you have to use a lot of learned techniques to achieve that end. Some of it is so unnatural for you and so high minded, that in order to achieve this state you have to play a role, for which you may or may not be equipped by nature. Furthermore you may have picked up, from the example of your coevals, or as a result of exposure to your fellow commuters through this aggressive world, habits of behaviour which are frankly inimical to the practice of good medicine. The less well equipped you are, the more you have to rely on training.

TYPE-CAST BY NATURE

In most countries young people have to choose to take up medicine by the age of sixteen. Although the best people keep on maturing until they die, so they are never really mature, at sixteen many are not mature enough to know whether they have got an aptitude for medicine. Fortunately there is an enormous range of jobs within medicine, from general practice through to being editor of a medical journal. Some people remain too shy, too uncommunicative, and not good at putting themselves in other people's shoes. It would be best if all these people could be put into, or would have the insight to put themselves into, branches of medicine which have little or no contact with patients. Unfortunately for them and for the patients, medical teaching is oriented towards producing doctors who treat patients, and as the rewards in gratitude and the satisfaction of doing good by direct action are so enormous, a number of doctors who are ungifted in the art of putting themselves over are tempted to stay with treating the sick. These doctors have to put even more effort into role-playing than their colleagues; and if they are good at the other aspects of doctoring then there is no reason why they should not be artful enough to do a convincing job. After all, the actor is not actually Hamlet; he is only pretending to be Hamlet.

PLAYING YOUR ROLE

You step into your role as a doctor as you leave for work, just as one steps into breeches and boots for riding a horse. You *can* ride in shorts, but nobody who is any good does. And when I say that you put on your kit, I am not referring to your white coat, although that does in fact help a lot; I mean that you say to yourself "Now I'm being doctor, which means doing those things which will promote the healing of the sick." And that is partly an attitude of mind, and partly a matter of observing Cab Calloway's dictum: "It ain't what you do, it's the way that you do it, that's what gets results."

LOOKING THE PART

The doctor should wear a proper attire. Just as modern dress obtrudes in Shakespeare's plays, a doctor's Hawaiian shirt, though it does not affect his knowledge, decreases his credibility; so does the smell of garlic or of a lunchtime beer; if an otherwise splendid doctor is dirty and unkempt he will be less effective; the surgeon who has cut himself shaving depresses the patient. Even if a single patient is put off, it is one too many.

The more junior you are, the less you can afford to dress as you please. When I was a student I used to wear a dark suit; I felt I needed it. The student must bear in mind that although "he's got to learn sometime," it is rather bad luck on the individual patient who has to be mauled about over and over again, by inexpert hands, often when he is feeling ill. The onus is firmly on the student to disturb the patient as little as possible and this starts with his appearance. A student in a crash helmet and a leather jacket may well be the best student in the class, but he is improperly dressed for the role of doctor. It is not enough to say "If I were a patient, I wouldn't mind being examined by someone in football boots if he knew what he was doing," because in the first place students may not know what they are doing, and in the second place it is the point of view of the most conventionally minded patient you could possibly meet who must determine the way you are to look. You should be dressed so that no one, no matter how conventional or contentious, could find fault with your appearance. The student must always bear in mind that looking at patients is a privilege, and that those with privileges have responsibilities.

It is true of course that the patient in a teaching hospital has the advantage of all the extra expertise that goes with these great institutions, and that because the students ask questions, the teachers have to think more about the patient in order to answer them. This may help the patient's treatment, as may the extra staff that teaching hospitals habitually carry. The student may be the patient's houseman at his next admission. The price the patient has to pay for these advantages is that he is "taught on"; but we must not make that price too high, and the patient must be able to feel that at least his student looks like a doctor.

Eccentric clothes and hairdos are to be avoided. If you need a model, try and dress like a bank manager. If you wear a white coat, it should be clean. Hairdos should not only not be eccentric, but the hair should be neatly groomed, and under control. Most people take exception to having lank, dank, dirty-looking hair drooping over them during an examination. Quite often such a hairdo is in fact clean, but this is beside the point. It is the impression which it makes on the patient that has to provide the guideline. Whatever you do out of the sight of patients is your own business, but when you are with them, or likely to see them, your standard should be that expected by the most conventional patient.

Patients tend to look at your hands as you touch them. You and I know that hands which have been repairing motorbikes all Sunday may have been washed over and over again and still be grained with oil on Monday. Once again, the patient's point of view must prevail, and such hands must be pumiced or washed in strong detergent or rubbed with carbon tetrachloride before the patient sees them. Nails should be kept groomed and at a length suitable to the bedside rather than to the boudoir. If you want to examine patients, you have to sacrifice long nails, however visually becoming they may be.

CONFIDENTIALITY

Walking about the hospital, or taking the lifts, you should not talk about patients, because the man standing next to you may be the patient's father, or more important, he may get the impression that you talk about people loosely. The doctor–patient relationship is a private one and you should never mention patients' names in public places. It is best not to mention their names even to your wife or husband, because it is a breach of confidence. I never tell my wife or family about our friends or acquaintances who consult me. It is best not to talk shop at all in the presence of laymen.

Careless Talk

It is important not to complain about or criticise colleagues or other departments in public. "This place is going to the dogs," shouted in a lift full of patients and their relatives, is not likely to inspire confidence in someone about to undergo a hip replacement. And almost everyone in a hospital is there because he or she is going to have something done, or is closely related to such a patient. The fact that it is your honest and well-founded opinion that it is actually going to the dogs is immaterial.

2. TAKING THE HISTORY

BEFORE CALLING THE PATIENT IN

The interview begins before you call the patient in.

The Referral Letter

General practitioners and medical students have to elicit all information from the patient himself. Hospital doctors usually have a letter of referral. Reading the doctor's letter is quite an art in itself. Very often the writing is illegible and when it is not, there is a very good chance that if he is consulting you, it is because he is stuck and up a blind alley. It is easy to get up the same alley yourself if you pay too much attention to what he says, so you have to read the letter but suspend judgement on it until you have seen the patient. You must also read it to see what drugs the patient has already had. Quite often the letter will ask some question about the patient which is not immediately relevant; if you do not read it until after the patient has gone, it may be too late to answer it and this is very annoying for the referring doctor. You must remember that you are treating the referring doctor too. If the letter of referral is a good one, I make a point of saying so to the patient. The letter should contain any relevant matter which the hospital doctor is unlikely to find out. Any relevant social or family or personal history which the patient may not divulge or which he does not know about should be mentioned.

Inadequate Referral Letters

Letters of referral are often unhelpful. Sometimes they long-windedly describe the symptoms and signs which you are bound to elicit yourself, but do not say what drugs the patient is having; and few patients know the name or the dose of the drugs which they take. Sometimes the doctor's letter contains a disparaging remark about the patient: "This patient is the most neurotic person in my practice." Patients will often open letters which their doctors give them, or they may get an opportunity to thumb through the notes in which the letter and other tactless remarks are filed. The more neurotic they are, the worse they take these remarks. And of course being neurotic in no way protects a patient from having organic disease. Nor should the doctor regard neurosis as less serious than organic disease.

Patients are often described as "cooperative" or "uncooperative." These are curious words to use when describing a patient who has, after all, come to consult you. Of course he is cooperative, unless you have upset him, in which case it is you who is not cooperative. I agree that the patient may be uncooperative when the umpteenth student has asked him the same question for the nth time, but part of the art of being a student is to woo the patient so that he becomes cooperative, and writing down the word "uncooperative" indicates that you have failed to adjust yourself to the patient in the way which good doctoring requires. Of course some patients *seem* uncooperative, but a good doctor can usually put an end to all that.

Refreshing Your Memory

If you are seeing a patient you have been treating for some time, you should read through the notes to re-familiarise yourself with his condition. The patient may be only one of thousands you treat, but as far as he is concerned he is the most important, and if he has seen you before he feels that you will know all about him. It looks bad if you greet the patient with "Well Mr. Smith, how did the operation go?" and he replies "I haven't had it yet doctor."

The long letter which is sent to the patient's general practitioner serves also to give you a summary of your thoughts about the patient when you saw him last. The letters should therefore all be kept together, in series, so that in reading through them you can familiarise yourself in a few minutes with the history of the patient's illness. From the letters you determine the purpose of the patient's visit, and this colours your approach to the interview. Of course patients do not expect you to remember tiny details, although they love it if you do and so it is acceptable to look at the notes to find out what blood group he is, or the date of his discharge from hospital. But if you cannot remember which kidney is affected, it makes the patient wonder if you have put him down for the correct operation, and the look in his eye tells you that you have dropped a point in the battle to send him out as happy and well as can be.

If a new doctor or a new student sees a patient on a return visit he should say to the patient early in the interview: "I've read your notes and I see . . ."

When the Notes Are Missing

However good one's memory, it is rather dangerous to see patients one has seen before if their notes are not available. Frequently the search for the notes has not been as diligent as it might have been, and the first line of attack is to institute a more thorough search, even if this means that the patient has to wait until the end of the clinic. Most patients would rather wait in these circumstances. If the notes still cannot be found, and the patient is unwell, or has come a long way for the consultation, it is often possible to treat him properly by a combination of questioning and re-examination. It is a mistake to convey to the patient either that you have not the faintest memory of him and his disease or that you remember every detail of his medical history. Whenever possible it is best to put off any change in medication until the notes have been found. A few patients carry lists of the drugs they are taking, or it may be necessary to telephone the patient's general practitioner, to get him to read back to you your previous letters about the patient. If there is no great urgency, you can tell the patient that he should go and see his general practitioner, who will prescribe something that the two of you have agreed on. If you are forced to take immediate action, and no information is available, you should prescribe that drug which is least likely to interact with any other drug, and which has the least number of contraindications. Successful treatment of the patient with lost notes is one of the hallmarks of proper doctoring.

THE PATIENT'S STANCE

Although the doctor is used to consultations, the patient is not and most are under stress. Bathed and in his best clothes, having rushed to get to the appointment on time, he sits outside the consulting room, desperately trying to get his story right, trying to remember, because coming to the consultation has of course banished it. He feels like a medical student does at his final viva.

When a patient feels ill, all sorts of thoughts pass through his mind which conspire to make his behaviour abnormal. The disease itself may affect his personality by altering his chemical or hormonal *milieu intérieur*. If he is in pain or deprived of sleep, his behaviour may change. If he has taken medicine to cure himself, this too may affect his personality. There are also many psychological causes for change in behaviour. The symptoms may prevent the patient from earning a living, or from coping with responsibilities. The fear that the disease may be serious, incurable or even lethal and the fear that the treatment may be unpleasant, are all extremely worrying. Some patients fear that no organic basis for their symptoms will be found and that they will be labelled as "neurotic." The list of psychological and organic causes for abnormal behaviour in sick people is extremely long.

In addition to all this, people's reaction to disease in themselves and in others is very primitive. A sick cow is jostled and kicked and may be killed by the herd, and this animal feeling persists to some extent in us, although it is overlaid with more civilised feelings of pity and compassion. These too may be quite hard for the sick patient to put up with for they are often more worrying than the disease itself. The patient may feel that by becoming sick he has failed, and this feeling may be greater now since the profession has started to belay the public with its recipe for positive health, than it was in the old days when disease was thought to strike like lightning, entirely at random.

These and many other reasons, combined with the peremptory way in which patients are treated in hospitals, mean that the patient arrives in your waiting room with the balance of his mind disturbed. By your manner and attitude you have to help him to recover his balance, and everything you do or say should be calculated to bring that about. Throughout the relationship you have to make allowance for the fact that the patient is being acted upon by forces which neither of you may recognise or understand, which may modify what he says and how he says it. You can only help the patient if you listen to what he says, observe how he says it, and what he does not say, and *relentlessly* try to get at what he really means.

Because the patient is not himself, you have to make full allowance for anything offensive or shocking which he might say. What a patient says may have to be taken as a manifestation of his disease, and should no more upset or disturb you than the statement that he is short of breath. If you are quick to take offence or lose your temper, you have to school yourself to accept anything which is said as a manifestation of disease, which cannot possibly be taken as cause for offence. If you take offence you do irreparable damage to the relationship.

I hope that by this time it is becoming clearer why acting the role of doctor takes as much thought and skill as acting Hamlet and that it is equally necessary to act in both situations.

THE DOCTOR'S STANCE

As a doctor, you take up a stance which will enable you to send the patient off as happy as and as well as is humanly possible. That is the minimum requirement; it is also close to the maximum possible result.

Being Nice to the Patient

You must be nice to patients at all times. Whether you like them or not, whether or not they have just come in from mugging old ladies, regardless of their record or their manners you cannot allow your personal view or feelings to come between you. It is a mistake to go to the other extreme and treat patients as friends, because the patient will feel that is forced and unnatural. One or two doctors do manage friendship, but this is a rare gift. Patients often "protect" the doctor by not telling him unpleasing facts, and if you become friends the patient may not want to hurt his friend's feelings by telling him that the treatment has not been effective. Although you will train yourself to accept the failure of treatment stoically, the patient will not know that; and unless patients reveal all the relevant details you cannot treat them properly. Treat patients as you would treat a stranger met in a friend's home.

I heard a Professor of General Practice telling students that if you do not like a patient, you should examine the reasons for your dislike and try to overcome it. Your reasons for disliking someone may be insuperable and the possibility of liking all the thousands of patients seen in a year seems remote. The amiability of patients has a bell-shaped distribution and some patients, like some doctors, are unpleasant. But a patient is not an unpleasant man with bronchiectasis, he is simply a man with bronchiectasis. His amiability concerns you only in those rare circumstances when it affects his treatment, and it occupies a negligible corner of your mind. You are not his wife or his son, you are his doctor. A professional approach to patients ensures that you are nice to them, and treat them as well as you possibly can; it is immaterial whether you like them or not.

Professional Niceness

If you are unhappy or tired or annoyed or feeling ill, you must not let it interfere with your performance. This is one of the reasons for role-playing. You put on your niceness with your white coat, and however horrid you are in real life, you pretend to that degree of niceness which is necessary for optimal results. Coldness, condescension, rudeness, brashness, arrogance, tactlessness or frivolity—even when combined with otherwise superlative performance—make for bad doctoring. Niceness is normally distributed, but we can all be nice when we want to. I doubt if anyone has been nasty while in conversation with the Head of State, and if you can manage to be nice to him, you must manage it for the patients. All the truly great men and women I have ever met have been nice, but we do not have many truly greats in medicine. The medium-greats are often not so nice. Perhaps they feel that careless arrogance and evident superiority will make them appear to be truly great.

Seeing patients and not being nice is analogous to a concert pianist going on to the platform with some of his fingers tied together. You can manage in a fashion, but you will not give a virtuoso performance. You are paid to be nice; if you do not feel up to it, a change of career might be the best solution. Being nice to patients is in itself quite an artful role. Professional niceness is not like the bonhomie of friends or the flirtatious relationship between attracted persons. It is neither unctuous nor overdone. It is serious and never joking, because to the patient his disease is entirely serious. Judicious levity from the experienced clinician, never at the patient's expense and with carefully selected patients, sometimes works wonders, but in general, if you are a bit of a wag it is best to save it for your colleagues.

Your stance should convey to the patient that you are there to help him and that you are pleased to do so.

Looking the Patient in the Eye

My hero, the late Dr. Geoffrey Evans, who was the best patient-handler I have ever known and on whose teachings much of the advice in this book is based, used to say that the jaw line revealed inheritance, the lips showed what life had done to the patient, and the eyes revealed the emotions of the moment. In order to convey your professional niceness you must look the patient in the eye, at the very beginning of the interview. Your eyes tell him what your stance is. If you wear spectacles, you have to work even harder to get the message through.

MEETING THE PATIENT

A Positive Therapeutic Presence

A proper doctor is all revved up and ready to cure before he calls the patient in, and as soon as he sets eyes on him he engages his first therapeutic gear. If it is clear that the patient is ill enough to require admission to hospital, while the doctor is saying "Hello" he is wondering if he has an empty bed. At this stage in the encounter he does not have the information for any more precise therapy. If he wonders how to evade his responsibility, or more forgivably thinks to himself that this means he will miss the first act of *Die Meistersinger*, he is not a proper doctor. Throughout the interview the proper doctor sniffs around for clues which will enable him to turn out a properly doctored patient. He sees the patient as a challenge, and seizes the opportunity to send him out feeling better than any other doctor could.

Calling the Patient In

Although many general practice surgeries are held in inadequate premises, the buildings are usually small and on the human scale. Large hospitals are a bit like cattle markets and there is an awful lot of ordering about, waiting, and being misdirected. The hospital itself, no matter how nice everyone is, and they aren't invariably so, is usually frightening as an institution, though you may not recognise this if you work in it. The patient may also be frightened of his disease and frightened of the treatment. You start to remedy all this as you get the patient in, if you address him or her as Mr. or Mrs. or Miss. Going to the door and roaring "Next" or "Robinson," is not only ill-mannered but helps to perpetuate the "anomie" or sausage-in-the-machine feeling that the patient is likely to have got before reaching you. Regardless of what he or she is used to at work—or even deserves (Shakespeare said "use every man after his desert and who should 'scape whipping")—everyone is entitled to a prefix to his or her name. It is particularly important not to call Mrs. Robinson, Miss Robinson and vice versa. It is your first therapeutic opportunity, and though tiny, it is too good to miss. It is particularly offensive to call the patient "Dad" or "Mother." If you cannot remember the name, say "Sir" or "Madam."

For several reasons I make a point of calling the patient in myself. Quite a lot can be learned from watching the patient cross the waiting area. If at the same time you note how many patients are waiting, it helps you to judge your pace. It also means that you are standing when the patient comes in, which helps to counteract the sausage-machine aspects of hospital visiting. It allows new patients to see what you look like before their turn comes. Getting up to call the patient in by name, with a handle to it, seems to me to be better medical and social manners.

Some doctors shake hands with their patients, and this early physical contact does reinforce the welcome. Some people are not enthusiastic about handshaking, however, and sometimes they seem more embarrassed than pleased by the outstretched hand. If the patient is escorted into the consulting room and his name is announced, it is more appropriate to shake hands, and if you rise as he enters and say "I'm Dr. . . ." and offer your hand, again it seems more suitable. You can try and estimate whether or not the patient wants to shake hands, and act accordingly. In some clinics, both in general practice and in hospital, the doctor reads the notes or the referral letter first, and then the patient is brought in by a nurse. This practice has the advantage that the nurse can introduce, or re-introduce, the patient and the doctor.

Greeting the Patient

You smile, say "Hello" or "Good morning" or something like that and ask the patient to sit down. If he sits facing you across a desk, the desk acts as a barrier between you. The patient should sit on one of two chairs placed at the side of your desk. The second chair can accommodate his belongings or it can be used by an accompanying person. If you are late, you apologise. Patients get annoyed if they are kept waiting, but are infinitely understanding if you excuse yourself.

I have seen doctors who do not look up from their writing, or point to a chair, or who allow the first moments of the interview to pass without saying anything at all. A smiling welcome is the first shot in the doctor–patient relationship, and it indicates that you are pleased to see the patient in the hope that you may be able to help him. It tells him that you are kind, efficient, approachable, likeable, expert, and that you have an all-out commitment to his welfare. It also tells him that you are not one of the dreaded band of doctors who regard patients as a nuisance, to be fobbed off, or who regard medicine simply as a means of earning a living.

Your greeting helps to put the patient at his ease. Your stance should tell the patient that your hobby is making him well. Solving a patient's problem as professionally as possible is as pleasurable as any other hobby, and when the time comes when you find Outpatients a trial, you should retire, or change to administration. The patient may be pathetic, grotesque, repellent, comical or attractive, and in each case the doctor's response must be professional. Whatever the patient's appearance or manner, the doctor's self-discipline should ensure that his response is appropriate. The ability to adjust to any patient is a hallmark of the proper doctor.

Checking on the Notes and X-rays

Sometimes a patient mishears and responds to the wrong name. For this reason it is advisable to welcome him by speaking his name clearly. Some patients are so excited by the prospect of the consultation that they mishear, and so it is important to see that the patient's symptoms are those mentioned in the referral letter, and that the patient's age and sex fit with those in the notes. Sometimes reports from special departments are filed in the wrong notes, and it is a good habit to check the patient's name each time you read such a report. The patient's notes may be accompanied by another patient's x-rays, or another patient's x-rays may have got into the folder. Each time you examine an x-ray you should start with the patient's name.

A Conversational Icebreaker

Some patients are desperately keen on getting down to hard facts, but many are set at ease by some preliminary, non-medical conversation. The weather, or the ease with which they got to the clinic, or something about their home town if they come from a distance, are suitable subjects for conversation. As you get more skilled in handling patients, you can ask where they come from, if they have an unusual accent or are obviously foreign, but these questions may give offence because the patient may interpret them as meaning that you resent having to see foreigners. Many patients dress up specially to come and see the doctor, and it is fitting that this very pleasing courtesy is acknowledged. You must ensure, though, that your comment is not seen as flirtatious or impertinent. Perhaps these things are easier for the older doctor to say.

Some doctors insist on all patients being stripped and lying on a couch before they meet them. This is a pernicious habit which promotes "anomie," increases embarrassment, makes the patient more vulnerable and deprives the doctor of much useful information.

TAKING THE HISTORY: WHY AND HOW

If you took a hundred consecutive patients and allowed one doctor to take the history but not to examine the patients, and another doctor to do a physical examination but not to talk to the patient, there is no doubt that the one who took the history would get the diagnoses right more often than his colleague. So, in order to achieve the best end result, you have to take a history, and as with everything else you do, you have to take a good history if you want to maximise profitability.

Be Interested

A good deal of "research" is being done into interviewing techniques, and the authors come up with some mind-boggling conclusions. In one such paper it states that the history-taker should appear to be interested in what the patient is saying. He should not *appear* to be interested, he should *be* interested. Interest in what the patient says is a basic minimum requirement. Lack of interest is incompatible with proper doctoring, and the student who has to simulate interest would be better employed doing something in which he *is* interested. What the patient has to tell you is pure gold, sometimes alloyed with a little make-believe, and it is absolutely fascinating. Your task is to extract from him every single fact and feeling which will influence diagnosis and hence treatment. This is a difficult task, and although it is more fun, at the beginning, to listen down a stethoscope, listening to the patient talking is a more profitable enterprise.

Medical students feel that they can learn more from patients with organic disease, preferably those with physical signs, but most patients, even in hospital, have no signs, and no organic disease either, so this is the "population" with whom you will be working.

Showing Off

Most people work best for the satisfaction they get from doing something well, and doctors are no exception. After a particularly brilliant coup it is difficult to restrain oneself from rushing out and putting it up on the hospital noticeboard. This feeling is right and proper, but there is a grave danger if you play to the gallery. The gallery may be the patient or the students or colleagues, but it is untherapeutic to do or say things in order to score points. There is only one safe way of showing off and that is letting your excellence speak for itself. Doing things properly, getting things right, maximising profitability, speaks for itself. Good wine needs no bush. There is no need for self-aggrandisement; high performance makes you grand enough. If I feel self-aggrandisement coming on, I divert it with a mental wink to Geoffrey Evans' ghost. Grandeur is a handicap in a doctor, and if you are cursed with it you will have to work much harder to get good histories. It may be some consolation that it helps when you are giving advice.

Hurry

Some doctors try to increase their stature with tricks. One of the commonest ways of doing this is to appear to be very busy. Hurry is the enemy of proper doctoring, and all the great men I have known seem to have all the time in the world for the patient or for their juniors and colleagues. The patient must feel that you have nothing on your mind except his problem, and that you will spend as long as it takes. That may or may not be a long time; if you rush the patient, it is bad doctoring. If circumstances force you to rush, you must contrive to do so without appearing to; make a note of what you have not had time to do, and do it at the next opportunity.

Interruptions

A telephone call from the French ambassador will impress your patient, but when you are taking a history there should be no interruptions whatsoever except for medical emergencies. The patient has to wait a long time for his interview. He has lots of things to tell you; he is entitled to your undivided attention. If you are interrupted, your concentration is broken, and medicine is too difficult a subject to be done with only part of the mind. Unless you are strict there can be a constant flow of interruptions from the telephone, from nurses, from secretaries, from colleagues and even from the tea lady. All of them must understand that you are not to be disturbed except for an emergency. Messages can always be delivered whilst the patient is undressing, or between patients. If you wish to make a telephone call, do it discreetly, between patients.

If you are interrupted, excuse yourself to the patient, and let your expression convey that whoever the visitor is, the visit will not displace the patient's problem from the forefront of your mind. Whenever possible ask the interruptor to come back later, and if this is not possible, make the interruption as brief as you can. When you return to the patient, do not say "Where was I?"

Questionnaires

A bad habit has grown up of putting a barrier between the doctor who makes the decisions and the patient. Sometimes this takes the form of a questionnaire which the patient is invited to fill in about his condition. A questionnaire cannot see the patient's face nor can it evaluate his tone of voice when he answers the questions. If the questionnaire is looked at, and there is no point in doing it unless it is, the answers may mislead. Most answers need a good deal of probing before they become useful clues, and the questionnaire is neither flexible enough nor subtle enough to effect the change. The doctor of course has a list of questions which he always asks about any symptoms, and a list of questions which he asks about the symptoms which the patient has not mentioned, but the value of the answers depends on how the patient answers them.

Hazardous Help

Ancillary workers, doing research, or social work, or trying to lessen the doctor's load, may see the patient before the doctor does. This firstly means that the doctor gets a second-hand impression, from the ancillary worker's notes, of what the patient said; and if he has not read them, it is quite likely that the patient will not mention the symptoms again, on the grounds that it is already in the "computer" and that the firm knows about it. If the ancillary worker responds untherapeutically to what the patient says, the patient may decide not to mention that symptom or view to the doctor. Patients learn from the questions one asks to give the "proper" answer. If you are asked three times in succession by three members of the staff whether the pain goes down your left arm, you tend to amend your story a little so that it does, especially if the three questioners look disappointed when you say it does not. Patients are very kind to us and are often very keen to please.

It is therefore important that the doctor who is going to take the decisions should be the first one to talk to the patient. You may have to be quite firm to ensure that this happens.

In the Absence of Dr. "A"

If the patient's general practitioner tells the patient that he is sending him to the great Dr. "A," it comes as a disappointment to the patient if he sees a young and inexperienced Dr. "B." As the GP's own opinion may be better than that of Dr. "B" he may well be affronted by the substitution. The absence of Dr. "A" may be unavoidable, in which case Dr. "B" must say in his letter to the GP that he saw the patient in the absence of his chief, and that he has discussed the problem with him. Dr. "B" must ensure that the patient sees Dr. "A" on his next visit to the hospital.

THE PATIENT'S STORY

Your Attitude to What the Patient Says

The patient lays most stress on what troubles him most, and it is important not to lose sight of the presenting symptom. If the presenting symptom is headache, and on examination you note anaemia, which the haematologists tell you is due to iron deficiency, you might then order a barium meal, and detect a peptic ulcer. If this responds to treatment and the bleeding stops, the anaemia will be cured. You may feel rather pleased with your performance, especially if the patient had no gastro-intestinal symptoms. However, the headache will be quite unaffected, and as the patient had not noticed either the anaemia or the ulcer, his view about your performance will be less enthusiastic than your own. So you need to make sure that you treat the symptoms.

Circumstantial Evidence

Patients frequently attribute symptoms to some life event. Old injuries, or smoking, or overwork, or "since the accident," or "since my father died" are typical "causes" of symptoms. *Post hoc* is not necessarily *propter hoc*.

Symptoms may not be due to the patient's most serious disease. If he presents with palpitation, and routine chest x-ray reveals a small, operable carcinoma of the lung, it would be wrong to waste time trying to cure his palpitation. That can wait until after he has had his thoracotomy.

Sometimes the presenting symptom is not the one which the patient is most worried about. The patient may find the symptom too terrifying to mention until later in the interview, or he may not be able to bring himself to mention it at all. If you suspect this to be the case, you may ask if there are any other symptoms that the patient has not told you about, or if there is anything else which worries him. If he still finds it impossible to talk about, he may divulge it when he knows you better. Many patients have symptoms for a long time before they seek advice, and it is useful to ask them why they have waited so long, because it may reveal some change in them or in the symptom.

Symptoms Which Have "No Organic Basis"

About half the patients seen in Outpatients have no organic disease. It would be more accurate to say that a percentage of them have organic symptoms which we fail to recognise as such. This leaves a large number with symptoms which have no physical basis that you can ever determine.

Some will be over-interpreting the odd aches and pains which flesh is heir to, but they do have an organic, if trivial from the doctor's point of view, cause. Almost everyone is either overweight or unfit or both, and especially in the second half of life the ill-used body, or the under-used body, gives rise to symptoms which do not amount to a disease, and do not affect function, but, like a door that squeaks every time you open it because the hinge needs a drop of oil, are annoying. For oil, read exercise in the case of symptoms. Minor ill-health is normal. Nine out of ten people feel that they are below average in physical well-being, and if the symptoms are worrying, they consult a doctor.

Other symptoms have no organic basis. If your father and three siblings have died of carcinoma of the rectum, at about the age you are now, it is all too easy to identify the odd twinge in the abdomen with the early symptoms that they had.

Symptoms with a Psychological Origin

The next group of patients have organic symptoms from psychological disease. There are many reasons why man's body acts in this curious way, a full discussion of which is outside the scope of this book, but I will give a single example. People who have a feeling of failure, from any cause, may translate these feelings subconsciously into organic symptoms. They, and their acquaintances, may find it more acceptable to attribute failure to disease. Finally, a few people make up symptoms, quite consciously, for an ulterior motive—from the schoolchild who needs an excuse to miss physical education, to the victim of an accident who is seeking to increase the compensation.

With experience, you learn to judge whether symptoms are appropriate or not. Whether the patient is consciously or subconsciously "making up" the symptoms, the point of history-taking is to get a correct assessment of the patient's story, simply in order to be able to apply an appropriate treatment. There is no place in doctoring for a moralising attitude. The patient tells you his story and you take it on the chin, without flinching or tut-tutting or eyebrow-raising. If he tells you he beats his wife, you take it with the same apparent calm as if he had said that he had indigestion. If you show surprise, or call him a rotter, he will either stop telling you things, or try and shock you by inventing even more awful stories, or he will feel reprimanded. That is not your job, and no matter how strongly you feel or how you yourself behave, you are not cast—in your consulting room—in the role of Judge, no matter what you are like at home.

Continuous Assessment

The assessment of the patient's story thus requires different procedural rules from conversation or discussion with friends. Whilst you listen to what the patient says with great care, you are at all times trying to assess it, in order to make a correct diagnosis in order to treat him.

HOW TO ASK QUESTIONS

All medicine is problem-orientated, so is all history-taking, physical examination and treatment. So, as the patient enters the room, and you notice that he is short of breath, you think to yourself: "I must find out from the story, the signs and special tests, why this patient is short of breath SO THAT I CAN TREAT HIM PROPERLY." That aim is best served if you encourage the patient to tell you all he knows; you ask him questions which amplify what he has told you, and you then evaluate what you have found out. It is not like conversation, because you do not give your own opinion about what the patient says until much later, if at all, and not on individual details of the story. It is not like legal examination because you are not trying to convict the patient, nor to paper over the cracks. As I have already said, it is not like judging. It is assessing. You must not let your good nature mislead you any more than you allow your censorious side to criticise.

Adjustment of Your Performance to Suit the Patient

Although by and large it is safer to play substantially the same role each time, because you have more than enough on your hands without adding unnecessary repertory aspects, you have to make minor adjustments in your performance with almost everybody. You take it slowly with unintelligent patients. You try harder to make the ill at ease feel at home. If you think that the patient may feel unwelcome, you positively discriminate in favour of the underprivileged and minorities, not by giving them special treatment but by doing whatever is necessary to send them away feeling better. To each according to his needs.

The Bell-Shaped Curve

One of the most useful concepts in medicine is that virtually everything is distributed in a roughly bell-shaped manner. Whether as regards height, weight, intelligence, pig-headedness or good looks, most of us are average, some of us are very much below average, some very much above. There is every gradation in between. Even things which cannot be measured are distributed semi-quantitatively in the same way. The adage "There's now't as queer as folk" is a comment on how far out the tails of the bell extend in both directions. Some patients are more than three standard deviations from the norm at either end of the bell, and through doctoring you come to realise the truth of that adage. This means that you have to accept all variations of human being, and have a stance which will suit them.

You may see as a patient a Nobel prize-winner, closely followed by someone from the other end of the intelligence scale. You must be able to adapt to deal with them both, whilst maintaining a stable position in the middle. Though all men are equal, some more equal than others, the doctor is consulted because of his special knowledge: the Nobel prize-winner comes in the same role of advice-seeker as the educationally subnormal. You must not be deflected from a properly therapeutic role by either awe of the one or pity for the other. Such factors as the patient's age and physical condition influence what you do, but nothing is more dangerous than varying your routine because the patient is too important, or too physically attractive, or used to teach you geography. Although you change your role slightly with all patients, the treatment which is right and proper is right and proper for everyone, regardless of their status.

Tone of Voice

Even the words "How are you" can be said in various ways. "How *are* you?" sounds as if you ask because you want to know. "How are *you*?" sounds as if you had not expected to see him again. "Howareyou" sounds social, and as if the only proper response is "Verywellthankyouandyou?" A grateful patient may respond with "I'm fine, thanks to you doctor" but this does not mean that he is symptom free. Everything you say has to be modulated, so that it is not misinterpreted, and so that you do not convey meanings which were not intended.

Quite often your natural tone of voice is quite unsuitable for taking histories. If your mode of speaking won you a reputation for brilliant cut and thrust, with no holds barred, in the university debating society, it will confuse patients who are not used to that sort of thing, and will antagonise the ones who are used to that sort of thing but when ill do not feel up to it. Some people speak so quickly, and some have such odd accents, that they are very difficult to understand. Few of us realise what our accent is like. A tape recording is usually stilted and distorted, but a consultation with a sensible friend might lead to the conclusion that a change of speech pattern might be therapeutic.

Some doctors put on an unnatural, stern tone of voice when talking with patients. If you sound like a headmaster interviewing a boy caught smoking pot, you will frighten some of the most interesting histories away. The "erring child" approach is antitherapeutic. Be gentle, it is more doctorly. Peremptory commands, though suitable for the football field, are untherapeutic! "Please sit down" is better than "Sit down." Both are improved with a smile. "Go in there and undress," never a pleasing prospect, is softened and improved by "I'd like you to ..." or "Would you kindly ..."

Terminology

Without going into boring linguistic detail, I would like to emphasise the importance of choosing the right words when talking to the patient about the history of his condition. A student started his presentation of a patient to Geoffrey Evans with the words "This case complains of ..." Evans stopped him and said "You've only said four words and you've managed to rob him of his identity and of his self-respect. He isn't a case, he is Mr. Murray, and he doesn't complain, he simply states what his symptoms are and bears them with stoic calm."

Some Aids to Fruitful Questioning

With skill and a proper stance, you make the patient feel progressively more at ease as the interview proceeds. Questions should be designed to get at the truth, and you will not do that if the patient is ill at ease. You look at the patient and by unspoken eye-language, and by the tone of your voice, you leave him in no doubt as to your therapeutic motive.

Blustering, bullying, "answer my question, yes or no" courtroom questioning is unfruitful. Nor is the "philosophical" approach any good. I once heard a patient tell a neurologist that the pain was like having red-hot needles pushed into his calf. "Have you ever had red hot needles ...?" his inquisitor riposted, and when the patient said that he had not, he pressed home his "advantage" and said "Well, how do you know then?" The patient was made to look foolish, and his resentment made him uncooperative. The neurologist was one up on the patient intellectually, and ten down on him therapeutically.

Patients are not there to be scored off. The grown-up physician does not need to score off his patients; as it is always antitherapeutic, he avoids it. The aim is to be one up on disease. If you feel unable to resist being one up on someone, ace your colleagues by getting the answer right. I have never had red-hot needles pushed into my calf, but I have a fair idea of what the patient meant, and so had the neurologist. He was being silly.

Putting the Patient Down

Most important of all, the patient must never be made to feel silly. In the competitive atmosphere of the university or in friendly banter, people pounce on foolish remarks or an unfortunate choice of words, and pull the speaker's leg about them. This is a perfectly healthy approach, and it helps to raise intellectual and conversational standards. With patients, such comments, or amused or despairing looks, have to be rigorously suppressed. If you ask a question and get an irrelevant answer, you must rephrase the question without batting an eyelid. Sometimes a patient will answer the "wrong" question. If, for example, you ask him how long he has had his cough, and he replies that it is worse when he lies down, his answer may be more helpful than if he had answered your question, and you seize on it gratefully.

GETTING THE ANSWERS

The value of asking questions can hardly be exaggerated. Quite often, when a patient's diagnosis has defied his own doctors, a clinician called in for a second opinion will solve the problem by asking one or two new questions.

Everything depends on the way you ask questions and the way they are answered; the value of the answers depends partly on the actual words used, and partly on how the question is asked and answered. A good clue can be rendered useless by improper questioning and failure to see what lay behind the answer.

An Opening Gambit

In his letter, the referring doctor may mention only the symptom which most interests or perplexes him and not the one which most troubles the patient. An opening gambit like "What can I do for you?" allows the patient to say what is troubling him, and in addition confirms the usual message that your smile of greeting was meant to imply, namely that you are there to help. Sometimes you get a flippant answer to this question, or to other questions. Do not laugh; the role of comedian is unsuitable for both patient and doctor. After a while you will formulate your own opening gambits, to suit the whole range of patients. You may say "Your doctor writes that you get short of breath when you lie down." Note, you do not say orthopnoeic, even if that is what the doctor wrote. You continue, "Will you tell me about this symptom from the beginning?," or "When were you last quite well?" The words used to describe symptoms mean different things to different people, and the first task is to establish what the patient means by the word he has used. The patient may be affronted and think that you are stupid if you ask him what he means by "indigestion," but if you ask him what the indigestion is like, he can paint his symptom for you. It may then be apparent that what he is describing is in fact angina. You should encourage the patient to tell you all about his symptoms in his own words, and without interruption, and when he stops, you question him about it.

Evaluating the Presenting Symptoms

You have to evaluate the history and quality of each symptom. To do this you have to ask a lot of questions about it. You ask when, and where, and how much, and is it getting better or worse, and do you get it lying down, or standing up, or watching the television, or when you are alone, or when you are busy, and on and on, worrying the symptom like a dog with a bone, until you feel you could paint a picture of it which would be instantly recognisable to the patient. The patient may leave out what he regards as irrelevant details which may contain the vital diagnostic clue; so you must ask if there is anything else, no matter how trivial, which is associated with the symptom.

Having exhausted the potential of the patient's principal symptom, you do exactly the same with his next most important symptom. As your first step in treatment is diagnosis, you will at all stages in the history-taking be striving to arrive at a diagnosis. At the beginning of the history-taking you are trying to find out which system is at fault. If the patient presents with shortness of breath you "diagnose" heart or lungs, followed a long way behind by neurosis or neurological disease, with the alimentary and genito-urinary systems unplaced.

If the patient reveals that the dypsnoea is accompanied by angina, the respiratory system is demoted to a lesser place in your interest. It is not possible to be equally interested in every symptom and sign, and, in addition, it would take hours to examine a single patient. Indeed it would be counter-productive to do so, because one needs to concentrate and avoid distraction by too much detail, and there is a risk too of the patient becoming bored or exhausted by the process. The effects of some diseases are not limited to a single system, and diseases such as sarcoidosis may give rise to manifestations in any system. It is more difficult to take a history in these circumstances.

Other Symptoms Referable to the Presenting System

Once the patient has been questioned about his presenting symptoms, you ask him about other symptoms referable to the same system, because patients often fail to tell you about all their symptoms.

If you get a positive response to a question, this unleashes another half dozen questions from you about how and when and where and how much, until you could paint that symptom too. You must ascertain which symptoms come simultaneously, and you must establish the order in which the symptoms developed.

Routine Questions About Other Systems

Finally, having asked about the relevant system or systems, you ask a number of set questions about all the other systems. It only takes a few seconds to ask "Are your appetite, digestion and bowels normal?," and if the patient says that they are, no more questioning about that system is usually required. If the patient's answer reveals malfunction of another system, it has to be gone into with the same thoroughness as the presenting symptom. The history which you elicit may bear little resemblance to that in the referral letter. Patients sometimes change the story, or the patient's doctor may have got hold of the wrong end of the stick. Try and reconcile the two, without undermining the patient's confidence in his own doctor.

Lists of Questions

That is the bare bones of history-taking, and the appropriate questions are outside the scope of this book. Most medical schools supply lists of questions to be asked. These lists are designed to be comprehensive for all systems, and it is not always clear to the students that you are not expected to ask every patient each question on the list. It would take several hours to ask all the questions, and the questionnaire approach is to be avoided as it is too mechanical, going too deeply into some things and not deeply enough into others. The questions should be learned by heart so that you have tools to extract any detail about any symptom. They are like a palette of colours which enable you to paint a portrait of the symptom.

Getting to the Bottom of a Symptom

It is easiest if the patient tells you about a symptom, allows you to discuss it with him until you could paint it, and then goes on to his second symptom and does the same. You should watch him while he is talking, and then break off and write down your interpretation of the symptoms. Often a single word, such as "angina," is enough. Writing between questions, or at the end of the interview, allows you to watch the patient's responses and allows him a space to consider what he has said and amend it if necessary.

If the patient wanders round and round his symptoms it may be difficult to pursue any one of them to its end. It is best not to interrupt if the patient changes to another symptom before you have quite finished with the last, because the patient's train of thought will be interrupted, and this gives him the feeling that he is being rushed. It often makes the patient forget what he was going to say. On the other hand, if you let him go on, it may make you forget what it was you wanted to ask, and you have to guard against that. Although the diagnosis may be obvious to you at a glance, or after the patient's first words, you must ensure that the patient feels that he has told you enough to allow you to come to an accurate diagnosis.

Popping the Question

The most valuable symptom is the one which the patient volunteers. Even that must not be taken at face value, but at least it is unsolicited, and other things being equal, it scores high. The next best symptoms are the ones you ask about, and the value of the answer depends on how you ask the question.

If you suspect that a patient with pain in the chest has angina, the fact that it radiates into certain areas is often diagnostic. If you ask if the pain goes down his left arm, nodding your head encouragingly, the patient may say "Yes" in order to please the nice doctor who obviously wants it to go down his left arm. It is much better to ask if the pain goes anywhere. If he says "Yes. It goes down my left arm," that is a valuable answer. If he says "No" you can ask if it ever goes down his legs—where angina never goes. He may then say that it doesn't go down his leg, but it does go down his left arm. The firm contradiction which follows such misleading questions provides a valuable answer. If he says that it does not radiate anywhere, you should then, and only then, ask if it goes down his left arm. He may say it does, and the answer, although less valuable than the previous answer, is worth something.

There are many reasons why the patient may not have told you at the beginning of the interview that the pain went down his left arm. He might have forgotten. He might have known that it was angina and thought that you would, like him, know that angina goes down the left arm. The chest element of the pain may have been intense, making the arm element seem trivial in comparison. He might have left it out in the hope that you would then say that it was not angina; he might have been unable to tell an actual lie although he was willing to tell less than the whole truth.

Asking Difficult Questions

A number of topics are embarrassing to patients. Others are embarrassing for the doctor, and some are embarrassing to both. An embarrassed patient may not tell you the truth, so that your attitude when you ask unembarrassing questions must prepare the ground for later, more embarrassing ones. It must be clear to the patient that you are not judging; that you are not trying to trick him into some sort of admission which will be damaging to him or to your opinion of him and that you are not prying. You evince no surprise at anything the patient tells you; nor do you look puzzled. The history-taking face just looks receptive.

Appropriate Responses

Even when you discover that a patient has a dreadful history or family history which moves you profoundly, you have to make sure that your response is the appropriate one. Not bland indifference, not floods of tears, but therapeutic. This takes sensitivity and judgement and experience. You ask your embarrassing questions in exactly the same tone of voice you use to ask about dyspepsia. You act as if this were a check-list; you convey that to you at least, the questions and the answers are no different in emotional content.

Some questions like "Do you cough up blood?" are, in fact, rather shocking to almost everybody, and if you rephrase it as "How much blood do you cough up?" it gives the impression that it is fairly normal to do so, and it is easier for those who do have haemoptysis to admit it.

The Truth About Alcohol

Alcohol consumption is another question which tends to embarrass, and to which underestimates are usually given. If you guess that a patient is a heavy drinker, you say "How many bottles of Scotch do you drink in a day?," and the patient replies "Only one doctor." If you had asked him if he was a social, moderate or heavy drinker, he would have said moderate. True consumption is usually twice what the patient says, plus half what the spouse says, divided by two.

Grading Symptoms

All symptoms have to be graded in your mind for severity. Mild, moderate, severe and gross—for short, grades one, two, three and four—is usually enough.

Some symptoms are difficult to grade. I used to ask patients whether their pain was mild, moderate or severe. They almost always said that it was moderate. If it was only mild, they were loath to admit it because you might think that they were "wasting your time," and few would admit that it was severe, presumably because they did not wish to appear to be making a fuss. You have to estimate the severity of pain partly from an estimate of the personality.

HOW AM I DOING?

Whilst peering at the patient in order to see what is the matter with him, you should be watching him in order to see what is wrong with yourself. People are normally distributed for insight, and normally distributed for judgement of what they see when they look inwards. The extent to which they examine other people in order to see what effect they are having on them, is normally distributed too. So is the amount they care about their effect on others. Most people consider themselves to be more insightful and caring than the norm, but performance suggests that those feelings are over-optimistic.

Many patients are critical of their doctor's performance, but these criticisms are unverifiable in the absence of an independent witness. It is clear, however, from watching consultants, registrars and students dealing with patients, that some performances are inadequate. I have, from time to time, pointed out to perfectly nice doctors that their patient was clearly upset by what they said, and this view has frequently been received with amazement. All establishments tend to be pleased with themselves and their performance. You have only to suggest a change in the curriculum or in the training of junior doctors, to be met not with criticism of the proposed change, but with surprise that any change is necessary. If this attitude is taken into the consulting room, it leads to the assumption that whatever you do is all right, otherwise you would not be doing it.

Video Games

The vogue for videotape recording of consultations is further evidence of how unconscious some people are of their own performance. The broadcaster Alistair Cooke said that it took him twenty years of practice before he learned to behave naturally in front of the microphone—and the video camera is even more disturbing. The patient too knows that he is being recorded and he behaves unnaturally. In this totally bogus set-up both "actors" will be on their best behaviour, and yet doctors who have seen films of their own performance say that they had not realised that the patient was upset, or that they used long words, or that they kept picking their nose. These doctors, clearly below three standard deviations from the norm of insight, observation and self-awareness, become enthusiastic advocates of videotaping. The worse you are, the more benefit you are likely to derive from such films, but it seems extraordinary that a doctor can reach maturity—or anyway seniority—without being able to tell whether he is upsetting a patient, and without being able to hear that he is using long, incomprehensible words.

Sailing Too Close to the Wind

In thirty years of practice I have, I regret to say, upset some patients. Although I cannot prove it, I believe that I have always been aware of these failures. The un-insightful will ask how I know. They only know that they have upset patients when someone tells them. Of course one cannot tell if it is not diagnosable, but you monitor the effect on the patient of everything you do and say. The minor signs of incipient upset tell you to change course, before you have done any damage, just as the expert helmsman responds to slight changes in the wind which the tyro does not notice. Patients are as different as doctors, and you should be examining their reaction to you all the time to see if you are being maximally therapeutic. Your stance is not "Gosh, that was rather well put," but rather, having anticipated the proper way of putting your question to this particular patient, you search for signs that it has not been untherapeutic. However gifted you are, practice will make you better.

It's Just Not My Day

If an airline pilot makes an error of judgement "because it's just not his day," he is the first to hit the ground when the aircraft crashes. This has a positive therapeutic effect on his performance which we are denied in the consulting room. Further, if the pilot's flying techniques alarm the crew, their complaints will ensure that he is grounded. This incentive to high performance is also lacking in the consulting room.

Role-playing enables you to perform correctly when you are tired or fed up. Your professionalism and self-respect demand it. The doctor who "can't stand Mondays" or who is "all right on his good days" has passed the age at which he should retire.

DIAGNOSIS

Prejudice, which means judging before you have the facts, is clearly a less good way of coming to conclusions than is judgement in full possession of the facts. In some professions, like weather forecasting and tipping the winners of horse races, prejudice is all there is. It would be of little interest to anyone to describe the local weather conditions after they had occurred. And when we listen to weather forecasts we bear in mind the fact that they are often wrong. The wise take an umbrella just in case. Scientists maintain that they reason inductively, from the known facts, but Karl Popper says that in reality they test hunches, which are really only prejudices.

In medicine you have to delve deeply into the system which is at fault if you are going to make a diagnosis. You have to start narrowing down your field of interest from the beginning. From the moment you set eyes on the patient you have to start coming to conclusions.

Spot Diagnosis

The term spot diagnosis usually refers to instant diagnosis of the patient's disease from some give-away visual symptom, recognisable across a room. A malar flush or protuberant eyes or a peculiar gait often reveals the exact pathological diagnosis. Like a detective, you should be on the alert for clues. Diseases are often difficult to diagnose, and hence to treat, so you cannot afford to ignore anything.

Face-Watching

As the face is the most conspicuous nude part of the body, generalised skin changes such as jaundice or cyanosis can be noted, usually more easily at a first glance than when you have got used to a patient's colour. There is a stomach ulcer face and there is a depressed face, but much more interesting than these faces which give you the diagnosis are the character and thought-reading aspects of face-watching.

The jaw, lips and eyes are the raw materials of facial expression, but the picture painted on our face is much more complex, and more revealing and much more interesting. They say that the face is the mirror of the mind, but it is more than that. It fits over the soul like a surgeon's glove, and the skilled observer can read it like a book. Actually, faces are more like diaries than books, and each new entry is etched on, often more precisely than in words.

Doctors must read patients' faces in order to find out what the patient is like, and to evaluate symptoms. Even when the patient is silent, his face is talking and may sometimes be signalling that he has something up his sleeve which needs letting out. When the doctor speaks, the reception of each word is registered on the patient's face, and a doctor who ignores this running commentary on what he says is a fool.

When the patient returns for a follow-up visit, I make a practice of trying to tell whether he is better or not before I actually ask him. I then find out whether I am right, and the experience helps me to judge the true state of affairs in those patients who for one reason or another do not tell me what they really mean. It is difficult to describe what it is about the face which reveals the state of mind. Features have something to do with it, but expression is much more important. Expression reveals the inner person. As Edith Wharton said, "The muscles of character lie close to the surface of feeling."

Obviously involuntary movements, lip pursing, screwing up the eyelids and brow furrowings help a lot, but the expression is much more than all that. I am sure that we do not look at any individual feature when we scan faces. We recognise expression, like we recognise our friends, by looking at the face as a whole rather than by examining say the nose or the ears separately. We see the signs, we know what they mean, but we do not usually know why they mean it. Character, personal history, and feelings are etched on the face in a largely inexplicable way.

The Patient Under Stress

The response to the stress of consulting a doctor is both adrenergic and cholinergic. As the situation is more frightening than infuriating a cholinergic response tends to predominate, and in addition the majority of people normally have a dominant cholinergic response. Either response produces major changes in behaviour and in physical appearance, and your initial assessment of the patient's character is more accurately an assessment of his character under stress. This estimate has to be updated as he settles down, and you should do anything you can to accelerate that process. You are much more interested in what the patient is really like than in how he responds to moderate stress, although this too is of diagnostic interest.

Learning to Look

Spot diagnosis should include diagnosing what the patient does, and what he is like, and if he is happy or successful or bullying or put-upon, by looking at him. A farmer said that one of his farmhands was a "good looker," for though illiterate and innumerate he could look at a field full of sheep and know which one was missing. All doctors should be "good lookers," and they should practice on every-one they see.

On a bus or train you should look at the passenger opposite and decide that he looks like a bank manager, or perhaps an accountant, although an accountant might look more prosperous. He looks fit, as if he takes regular exercise. He looks as if he is a happy person, and can cope. He looks as if he is going to get off the train at Leamington Spa. Of course if you then note from peeping at what he is reading that he is a member of Equity and he gets off at Stratford-upon-Avon, you have to revise your initial estimate. You learn by your errors. When I get no confirmation from his reading matter or conversa-tion with his companion, I often yield to the temptation to lean over and ask him if he is a publisher, born in Huddersfield. When you get it right, the effect is dramatic, and I feel that though slightly imper-tinent, it is for the general good if it makes me a better doctor.

Diagnose everything, day and night, even whether the driver of the car ahead drives as if he will turn right without giving a clear indication of intent. And check up on your diagnosis whenever you can. Constant monitoring is the key to improvement. Geoffrey Ev-ans was once being driven at a snail's pace in a hired car. He asked the driver if there was anything wrong with the car, and when the man said no, Evans thought to himself that if it was not the car, it must be the man. "Do you drive the hearse?" he asked, and of course the man did.

Ceaseless diagnosis and observation of human nature are needed to enable you to understand people. Most doctors are middle class and have led sheltered lives. You cannot treat patients properly unless you understand them and the way they tick. The proper study of physicians is man.

Diagnosis from the Word Go

The patient's manner and appearance, distorted as it is because he is in the patient role, starts off in your mind the diagnostic process. The patient looks ill or worried, or fit and at ease. The patient looks complaining or stoical. The patient looks entirely trustworthy, or like a man you wouldn't buy a second-hand car from. The patient looks as if he would enjoy telling you all his symptoms down to the most trivial detail. The patient looks so self-effacing that he will not want to "waste" your valuable time by telling much.

The patient may also be unwilling to tell you certain things in the presence of a nurse or students or another doctor. This is one very good reason for seeing patients on their own. The presence of students, a necessary evil, impedes the doctor–patient relationship, because the patient is often inhibited—or worse, plays to the gallery —and the doctor's attention is divided—or worse, he plays to the gallery. Students and ancillary workers should sit in silence, at a distance from, and out of the sight line of, the patient. They should not crowd him in.

Fitting the Diagnosis to the Findings

You have to make up your mind what the patient is like, and adjust your technique accordingly. You assess his anxiety level because anxiety distorts him. It is worthwhile asking patients if they are regarded as an anxious person by their spouse. If you feel that the patient has not told you something important, you have to set about winkling it out by other methods, on your own, or later when you know each other better. Like the weatherman, you have to update your guestimate constantly. The prejudiced approach is extremely dangerous unless you are prepared to abandon your guess when it seems to be wrong. If you stick to your original opinion in the face of the facts, you are not a proper doctor.

Intellectual Honesty

The only thing which pays dividends in the long run is getting the treatment right, and the way to do that is to get the diagnosis right, and the way to do that is to abandon your preconceptions as soon as you find they do not fit the facts. If you have made a terribly clever spot diagnosis you may be tempted to cling to it, bending the symptoms and physical signs a little to force them to fit, just for glory. But it is a mistake; proper doctoring demands total intellectual honesty. There is more than enough glory in getting it right.

"DIFFICULT" PATIENTS

The Talkative Patient

Some patients are so talkative that unless you keep stopping the flow you never get to the bottom of the symptom. Although you appreciate that the patient is lonely and needs someone to talk to, some line has to be drawn, as it is not practicable to spend the whole day talking to the lonely.

Some neurotic patients seem to be testing the doctor's stamina. They go on and on, with one complaint after another, and no matter how long you keep going, they always seem to have further symptoms to mention. Regardless of the amount of time you have spent they seem to be just as upset whether you terminate the interview early or late. On occasion, I have decided to let one of these patients go on until they stop. I have never managed it, and I have a feeling that they want you to lose your patience with them. Then they can tell their family that "He never listens."

There is really no satisfactory way of cutting a patient short. He knows that you have a waiting room full of patients and that the end of the clinic is approaching, but he cannot bring himself to accept his fair share of the time available. If you say that you have fifteen more patients to see or that you have spent half an hour already and that you have not examined him yet, he gets upset. The lightest response, even a nod of the head, licences the patient to unleash another flood of symptoms. If you feel that you really must end the interview it can be done, with least offence, if you say "Thank you for giving me such a full story. Perhaps you could get undressed now so that I can examine you." I suppose in one's private consulting room one might press a hidden button to signal one's secretary to phone, and after a brief spoof conversation, pretend that the patient had finished talking just before the telephone rang. In the extreme case, taking the temperature with an oral thermometer may be the only solution.

"I'm Sorry to Have Wasted Your Time Doctor"

Patients often apologise for wasting your time. Almost invariably it is the ones who are not wasting your time who apologise, and I always strenuously deny it, and tell them that I am paid to listen to people. The patient has no way of knowing whether he is wasting your time or not, unless he is malingering and malingerers never apologise. Indeed, the longer they talk, the more certain the diagnosis becomes, so even then the time is often not wasted.

Maladie du Morceau du Papier

The occasional patient produces a piece of paper on which he has written all his symptoms or all the things he wants to ask you. For some reason which I have never been able to fathom, this produces curious responses in some doctors. They either regard it as a joke, or they get annoyed. Two doctors talking in a features programme on radio agreed that the piece of paper was the thing which annoyed them most about patients. Not everyone is gifted with a good memory, and in the excitement of the consultation the patient is likely to forget to say or to ask something. What could be more reasonable than to write it down?

"I Have Shy–Drager Syndrome Doctor"

Patients occasionally tell you the name of the disease from which they suffer, and some doctors get annoyed when told, as if the patient had somehow spoiled things by this premature revelation. Everything the patient says must be accepted as potentially useful information, which has to be evaluated. Nothing which the patient or the referring doctor says is taken at face value, and any diagnosis he offers is subjected to a flood of further questions in order to determine whether or not it is correct. Confirmation of what the patient says should be sought from the doctor who made the diagnosis.

Silly Patients

When we describe behaviour as silly, we mean that it is unsuitable to a person of that age, intelligence, common-sense and judgement. Almost everyone does something silly from time to time, but some unfortunates are silly most of the time. Although silliness lies in the eye of the beholder, each individual doctor will have to deal with patients who he considers to be silly. Sometimes the silliness is due to embarrassment, and this will wear off with time and good doctoring, but every now and then you meet patients who are silly by nature or by habit, and they are difficult to deal with. More will be said about this in the chapter on giving advice (Chapter 7), but silliness does make history-taking difficult. It demands patience, extra firmness and seriousness, and self-control. Its reward is that it is more of a triumph when you succeed in extracting a proper history.

The Patient Who Cries

Sometimes a patient will break down and cry while giving a history. The doctor must on no account try and stop the patient crying, for the crying may be the best part of the treatment. You continue taking the history when you can, and you accept the crying as if all patients cried during history-taking. It often helps the patient who cries if you reach out and touch his hand or shoulder. If you are highhanded, bossy or offensive, a lot of your patients will cry during history-taking. I hope it has been made clear that these attitudes are unacceptable, although you may, with advantage, let a little more of your bossiness show when you give the patient your advice. All advice should be given at the end of the interview. It is a mistake to give your opinion about things as you go along, even though the patient asks for it. If he does, tell him, uncensoriously, that you would like to complete your examination before you give your opinion.

CHILDREN

There are a number of differences between adults and children which necessitate changes in the doctor's technique. Children are likely to be more apprehensive than adults. Their experience of life and of medical matters is not large enough to enable them to estimate whether the visit to the doctor is likely to be painful or not. An adult with a skin rash knows that the examination and treatment are most unlikely to be painful or embarrassing. A child will not know, and indeed a rash will inevitably involve an examination of his pharynx, which may well be unpleasant. In general, an adult patient has the experience to judge when he is suffering from minor illness, or when he may have some more serious disease, and adjusts his anxiety accordingly—a child cannot do this. These differences do not arise because the child is less intelligent than the adult; he is simply lacking data and experience.

If a child has had an unpleasant experience with a doctor in the past, he is likely to assume that all consultations are unpleasant. Some parents use the doctor or doctors in general as a threat and the child may feel that you will punish him. In a hospital corridor I heard a mother tell an erring four-year-old that if he did not behave, she would get the doctors and nurses to cut him up. If a child looks suspiciously at you, it may be because his previous experience with doctors has been unhappy or it may be because he believes that you are going to cut him up. You have to work very hard to reassure him.

For all these reasons, children are likely to be more anxious than adults, and the doctor has to modify his performance when dealing with them. In an attempt to get children to associate doctors with pleasantness, I "chat them up" when I see them in hospital corridors or lifts.

As a child is so much more dependent on his family than is an adult, the role his family plays both in the genesis and the treatment of his disease is even greater, and this means that a much deeper enquiry has to be made into the family relationships. The family history, the antenatal history and the developmental milestones of the patient play a larger part in diseases of childhood than in those of adults.

Ancillary Staff

Most people are nice to children, but it is very important that *everyone* who sees the child before he is seen by the doctor should be nice to him.

Waiting

Children have less patience than adults and it is best if they are seen as soon as possible after arrival, even if this involves queue-jumping. Children are often noisy and difficult to control if they are kept waiting, and the noise disturbs both the doctor and the other waiting patients, so it makes sense to see them quickly. Toys or games should be available in the waiting room for entertainment.

Welcoming the Child

Make certain of the child's first name and sex before you call him in; you can break the ice by asking him if he likes being called James or Jimmy. It takes more skill to welcome and gain the confidence of a child than it does an adult. Adults are usually keen to get on with the consultation and prefer a minimum of small-talk. You gain the confidence of children if you talk to them socially and unpatronisingly. Many students and doctors, particularly those without children of their own, are unable to think of any conversational gambits, and it is well worth thinking up some few remarks which will make a conversation, rather than a lecture.

Talking to Children

Children are always pleased if you treat them as serious persons, and your conversation should always be sensible. If the child thinks that you are silly, you will not get his confidence. Many people talk to children either in "baby language" or as if they were of low intelligence and this is a mistake even if the child's parents talk to him in this way. The child cannot talk about things which are outside his experience, but for those things which he knows about, his opinions are valid and interesting within the framework of values of his age group. Indeed, some young children will reveal astonishingly astute opinions if they are encouraged to talk. When in doubt, talk "up" rather than "down."

There is a fine line between adapting your conversation to the child's experience, and talking down. Most children will be shy and not at their best when you first meet them, and if you pitch your conversation too high, you will embarrass them and harm the relationship. Your effect on the child must be carefully monitored and you change course before you do any harm. It does not matter if you use the same conversation for each child, as long as you do not say it all over again on the child's next visit. Children, like adults, enjoy being the centre of attention and if you woo them in this way they enjoy coming to see you.

Playing with Children

Whereas the relationship with adult patients is always entirely serious, a child will often respond to a playful approach, particularly if he is feeling well. The level of play must be kept under control, particularly with boys, for if discipline breaks down the child may be unwilling to sit or lie still while you examine him. Children love to play with "new" toys, and stethoscopes, spatulas and plastic syringes are usually well received. It is best to offer disposable or dispensable toys, because children frequently do not like to give them back. If you allow a small child to draw with a pencil and paper, you can often make conversation about the drawing. A good deal can be learned from watching the child at play, both about his development and the effects of the disease.

Taking the History

Children are usually accompanied by an adult, and when they are very young this clearly is necessary. However, the doctor must remember that his first duty is to the patient. The parents are second. As soon as the child can answer questions, these should be addressed to the child, and the parents can expand the answer if they wish. The child must be left in no doubt as to where the doctor's allegiance lies. If you get the parents' confidence, by listening carefully to what they say, the child will see that what the doctor says has the parents' approval. You do not curry favour with the child, but you are as much on his side as justice and mercy will allow.

If you feel that the parents are spoiling the doctor–patient relationship during adolescence, you may have to let the parents see that from your point of view, although your behaviour toward them is impeccable, that their continued presence is unhelpful. You do not say so directly at first, but you address yourself entirely to the patient, and if the parent says something, you ask the patient whether it is true or what they think about it. Most parents get the message after a while, but occasionally you may have to put it into carefully chosen words, in a tactful tone of voice. You may have to look after a child for thirty years, and mishandling at the beginning may never be reparable. If the child goes into a cubicle to undress, the parents should go with him. If you allow them to stay behind, the child will think that you are talking about him behind his back. If either the parents or the doctor have something secret to say it should be said when the child is unaware that parents and doctor are in communication.

THIRD PARTIES

The Patient's Friend

Sometimes patients will ask if it is possible for their spouse or a friend to come into the consultation with them. The patient may actually desire the spouse or friend to be present, or he may have been coerced into pretending that he does. He may have been unwilling either for the "good" reason that the spouse is coming between him and good doctoring, or for "bad" reasons; for example, the patient may be unwilling to tell the doctor something which the doctor really should be told. If the patient has misrepresented the doctor to a spouse, the lie may be revealed if the spouse attends a subsequent consultation.

Whether the reason is good or bad, a practical compromise is to see the patient alone first. This gives the patient a chance to tell you anything which is strictly between the two of you, or to say "Don't tell my husband about..."—and it is astonishing what sorts of things they want to keep secret. It also demonstrates to both parties who your primary loyalty is directed to. The spouse or friend can be helpful if they confirm or deny the patient's story, or if they have observed an attack during which the patient suffered impairment of consciousness. As with parents of children, the spouse or friend should be sent in to "help" the patient undress. If this is unsuitable for one reason or another, the friend should be asked to wait outside until the patient has been looked at, and is back in the consulting room. If the friend is banished during the examination it gives the patient a further opportunity to say anything which is not for the friend's ears.

Interpreters

If the patient cannot speak English well enough to give a clear account of his symptoms, it may be necessary to use an interpreter. This is rarely entirely satisfactory and is commonly misleading. The patient may bring a friend or relative who understands very little more than the patient and this is often worse than useless. It is one thing to be able to order food in a restaurant, and quite another to be able to describe symptoms. Sometimes the interpreter is of a higher social class than the patient and if he is an official, say from the embassy, his attitude may be that his valuable time is being wasted describing this peasant's boring symptoms.

Interpreting the Interpreter

Interpreters frequently do not ask the question you ask, and you should listen to the translated question to see that it has roughly the same number of words in it that your question had. You may notice that the interpreter says the same four or five words to the patient, no matter what question you ask. He is actually saying "Don't worry, it won't hurt," and making up what he feels is the correct answer. Interpreters who are medically trained are often the most misleading of all because they try to interpret what you and the patient are saying, instead of just translating it. If you feel that the interpreter is doing badly, you may be forced to ask him to translate every single word that you say, and then you say three words at a time, and wait for them to be translated. This sometimes works but it usually infuriates the interpreter. Working through an interpreter no matter how well he speaks the language, deprives you of the nuances of the patient's history. Though it provides an insight into the difficulties under which vets work, it is not productive of proper doctoring.

CONFIDENTIALITY

There is no symptom, real or imagined, which, if reported to a third party, may not be used to the patient's detriment by some malicious or gossiping or overprotective person. Because of this, no one but the doctor should know about Mrs. Jones' cancer or bronchitis or anaemia, nor even that she had a splinter in her finger. Unhappily the clinic is often full of people who can see and hear what is said. There are the nurses, the students, the social workers, the clinic clerks and a host of other people who have both the opportunity and the right to look at and through the patient's notes. Although it is reasonable to leave anything clearly damaging out of the notes, what appears to everyone as not damaging may cause the patient to lose a job, or an opportunity, or even to be the subject of unwanted solicitousness by his friends and workmates.

Population Studies

In addition to what one might term the necessary overexposure of the patient's private affairs, there is the reporting of the patient's name and address and diagnosis for statistical purposes. It is of course necessary to collect statistics, if only to allow the epidemiologists to have fun with figures, but I cannot see why it is necessary to include names and addresses. The hospital number would do just as well and no one would be able to recognise the patient. The system of reporting patients was brought in when I was a registrar, and it was my job to fill in the appropriate form and the code of the diagnosis. There was a code for "Not yet diagnosed" and I filled in all my patients under that heading. This maintained privacy, saved time in looking up codes, satisfied authority, and the only one who suffered was my chief, who might have appeared to some studious bureaucrat to be incapable of diagnosing anything. I felt that his shoulders were broad enough to enable him to bear the load. One cannot of course control leaks from other sources, but one can ensure that one is not the source of a leak oneself.

Part of the Hippocratic Oath which all doctors have to swear, demands secrecy, and although it is increasingly difficult to maintain it, and although a judge may order a doctor to tell him something in breach of that oath, it is best to act as if the oath were absolute. This demands constant vigilance, and it is one of the many aspects of doctoring which calls for self-discipline.

WRITING UP THE HISTORY

Anyone who has tried to reconstruct a patient's history from the notes will know that, for the most part, notes are quite inadequate. Students are trained to write everything down, usually excessively long-windedly, but admission to the Medical Register seems to result in an untoward brevity. The shortest notes I have ever seen were "H.P.C. Rides a bicycle. Rx Dig." There was no referral letter either. You might say that it was perfectly clear what was in the doctor's mind, but the notes and the referral letter between them should enable you to say at a later date what the patient's condition was like, what the physician thought was the cause, and what action he took.

PAST HISTORY, FAMILY HISTORY AND SOCIAL HISTORY

Past History

In response to the question "Have you had any serious illnesses?" a patient may give an incomplete list. He may forget; he may not have realised that an illness was serious; or he may be unwilling to reveal a past history of say venereal disease, or of mental illness, which some people regard as shameful. If you then ask him "Have you ever had ... ?," offering a list of diseases which are relevant to his symptoms, you will jog his memory, and he may find it easier to admit to some "shameful" disease than he did to proclaim it before its name had been mentioned. Geoffrey Evans' lists of diagnostic questions to patients were famous. They usually began with an enquiry into any past history of "tonsillitis, quinsies, sore throats, glands in the neck, asthma, hay fever, bronchitis, pleurisy, pneumonia" and proceeded with grim determination through the alimentary system, ending with "typhoid, dysentery or yellow jaundice." A rather surprising one on trauma ended "Have you fallen on your back, fractured your skull, dislocated your spine, broken your neck—*much*?" If the disease of which the patient is ashamed is not relevant to his present symptoms, there is no point in stirring up distasteful memories simply to make the record complete.

Sometimes a patient has been misinformed about the nature of a previous illness, either deliberately or because the diagnosis was wrong, and the diagnosis should not be taken at face value. Questioning about the symptoms and the treatment which was given allows an assessment to be made of the correctness of the previous diagnosis. Wherever possible, confirmation should be sought from the doctor who treated the patient at the time.

Family History

Some diseases run in families, and there are two reasons for enquiring about that. The first is that one may be interested in, or trying to establish, the pattern of inheritance, or the purpose of the enquiry may be to assess the suitability of parents for further pregnancies. In these circumstances, it is necessary to enquire about the family history even if this distresses the patient. To ask these questions and to maintain a properly sympathetic attitude, which does not increase the patient's distress, calls for a good deal of skill.

The second reason for enquiry into the family history is that the patient may be presenting with the symptoms of the disease which affected his relatives. His anxiety that he has the same disease will be high, and discussion of the number and relationship of his family who have had the disease will serve to increase it. The genealogical instinct is a strong one, and those family trees which show the affected members have a fascination. But probing into bad family histories should be limited to those patients in whom the probing will be of practical value to the patient. In my opinion a statistical estimate of the likelihood that the proband will develop the disease does not have practical value in the individual case. This does not mean that the disease has to be glossed over or ignored, but like all unpleasant procedures the cost of persisting has to be weighed against the advantage to the patient. If the referring doctor states that the patient has a bad family history of such-and-such a disease, it is usually unnecessary to refer to the matter until the time comes for advice and reassurance.

Social History

The more long-term and incapacitating the disease, the more it is necessary to enquire about the patient's job and home, and about his way of life, his self-sufficiency and his supports. Tact, and limitation of the enquiry to what is germane to the welfare of the patient, should guide the questioning.

3. EXAMINATION OF THE PATIENT

HISTORY-taking and examination cannot be rigidly separated because the patient is observed for physical signs of disease from the moment he steps into the consulting room, and frequently, during examination, you will note a scar or a lump or some other abnormality which the patient has not told you about, and which you will have to ask questions about. The patient may tell you about another symptom while you are examining him, and you will have to question him about it before you can proceed with the examination.

The process of diagnosis is analogous to the procedure used to examine a slide under the microscope. You hold the slide up to the light to identify the part of interest. You then examine that part under the low power, and having got it into focus and into the centre of the field, you switch to medium power, centre, focus again, and finally change to the highest power. If you had started with the highest power it would have taken hours to find the right spot, and you might have damaged both the microscope and the coverslip in the process. Similarly, history-taking allows you to get the system which is at fault into focus, physical examination represents a more intensive look at a smaller area, and special tests are the oil immersion of data collection. The data are collected neither randomly nor routinely, but thoughtfully. On-line processing by the mind ultimately turns data into treatment.

By the time that you have finished history-taking, you will usually have diagnosed which system is at fault, and in physical examination, as in history-taking, you concentrate on the system at fault, because it is neither practicable nor advisable to go over everything with a fine-tooth comb. A curry-comb has to do for the "normal" systems. The word examination implies careful inspection, and careless examination is a contradiction in terms. If you are quite certain that the patient has no symptoms referable to the central nervous system, and if you have asked him your standard CNS questions, you will prepare yourself to give him a brief, but not cursory, examination of that system, having devoted the greater part of your time and mental energy to the system at fault. It is as though you can only focus entirely, with maximum energy, for a short time on each patient, and you want to reserve your peak performance for the most important part. Willie Sutton, a celebrated American criminal, when asked why he kept on robbing banks replied "Because that's where the money is!" Sutton's Law applies in medicine, and the doctor's time is most profitably spent "where the money is."

PREPARING FOR THE EXAMINATION: PUTTING THE PATIENT AT EASE

Nudity Is Embarrassing

Sometimes the examination couch is in the consulting room itself, and if so, it should be screened off from view. People who are fairly happy to be examined unclothed do not like being watched while they undress. All observers should absent themselves until the patient is actually lying on the couch, because people prefer not to be seen moving in the nude and certainly not until they have got used to being looked at while lying still. The "poetry in motion" aspect of movement in the nude is confined to the first twenty years of life, and that is the time of maximum shyness.

Although doctors are used to nudity, patients are not at all used to it. Public schoolboys, servicemen and showgirls tend to be less self-conscious, but the vast majority of people feel very uncomfortable when they are undressed. One might think that modern bathing costumes would have removed this shyness, for they leave little to the imagination, but the vestigial ribbons of cloth somehow preserve dignity. A dressing gown should be available and the patient should be asked to undress and put it on. It is embarrassing, cold and lowering to be made to lie nude on a couch. By using a dressing gown or a blanket, only the part which is being examined needs to be exposed. If a woman patient is to be examined while standing or moving about, she should be asked to put her bra on.

People feel protected, as indeed they are, by clothes, and the clothes are part of the persona which they present to the world. They also cover up a multitude of skins, many of which we would rather not reveal. The patient *must* be undressed; Dr. Cooke of Oxford used to say "Medicine with the clothes off is difficult; with the clothes on it is impossible." But it is the doctor's job to make sure that embarrassment is reduced to the minimum.

Helping the Infirm

Whenever possible, the infirm should be helped to undress. It is more satisfactorily done by a nurse—they are so much better at it, and some patients are embarrassed if the doctor helps, because they feel that it is beneath his dignity. If there is no nurse you should help the patient yourself, demonstrating, by your manner, that it is not at all below your dignity. Some people do not like being helped, even when they need it, and the help you give must be carefully titrated against necessity. You can also learn about the patient if you watch him coping with undressing. Small children should be undressed by the parent, even though fathers often make a worse job of it than the doctor.

Patients You Find Attractive

The consulting room is an unlikely setting for thoughts of a romantic nature; both patient and doctor are usually preoccupied with illness. Nevertheless, from time to time a doctor is attracted to a patient, and a patient may feel attracted to the doctor. In either case the feeling may or may not be reciprocated. Medical ethics forbid any development of the relationship, but what is more important, because it is commoner, is that the doctor must not let his feelings modify his behaviour. You observe that the patient is attractive just as you would observe that he had an upgoing toe, and your face and manner must be unaffected. Flirting with the patient, or allowing the patient to flirt with you, although within the letter of the law, is outside its spirit, and erodes the basis of proper doctoring.

Chaperones

It was formerly universal to have chaperones for patients, but with the shortage of nurses this habit has fallen into disuse. Theoretically it is advisable to have someone of the opposite sex, either another patient or an auxiliary, within earshot in case the doctor assaults the patient, or in case the patient claims to have been assaulted. As the incidence of alleged or actual assault is so low, and as there is often no alternative to examining the patient out of earshot—especially in domiciliary practice—this custom too seems to be falling into disuse. But whenever possible it is best to have someone else within earshot, and in what might be called "high risk cases," where either the doctor or the patient constitutes the high risk, it is advisable to have someone nearby.

The Examination Couch

Although many examinations have to be made in patients' homes, where adjustable couches are not available, in consulting rooms they should be standard, because the sick patient may be unable to lie flat. Furthermore, the position of the patient is often a critical point in the detection of physical signs. The cardiovascular system, for example, is best examined with the patient lying semi-upright, at 45 degrees; the abdomen should be examined with the patient almost flat; and examination of the femoral arteries is sometimes only possible with the patient absolutely flat.

Sometimes the patient cannot achieve these various positions, and then the efficacy of examination may be impaired, but it is usually possible to achieve a compromise position which is acceptable to both parties. It may be clear from looking at the patient that he will not be comfortable lying down, and then the doctor should adjust the couch so that the patient can lie comfortably, before the patient undresses.

The couch on which the patient is to lie, often against bare skin, should be covered with paper, which is changed after each patient. At the very least the head end should be fresh. Dr. M. B. Matthews installed an electric blanket on his examination couch, on the grounds that anxiety makes people feel cold, and that further cooling is unacceptable. The difference between a patient's dismay at the chill, and pleasure at the unexpected warmth, was for him one of the simple pleasures of practice.

Unnecessary Delay

The patient should not be left waiting for the examination any longer than is necessary. The bad habit of seeing two patients at a time in adjacent examination cubicles, besides dividing the doctor's attention—and from time to time confusing him—makes people wait too long before they are seen. Their tension mounts, and they become progressively more unlike themselves. If, as for example in patients with hypertension, you wish them to rest for a while before you measure their blood pressure, you explain that you are going to keep them waiting because it provides better readings; they then expect a delay, although they don't necessarily remain calm, and the blood pressure may actually rise. The occasional patient is claustrophobic, and you should be aware of this possibility.

THE DOCTOR'S STANCE DURING THE EXAMINATION

Examination is part of the treatment, and the doctor's approach to it must be positively therapeutic. From the way you set about the examination it must be clear to the patient that the niceness, interest and skill which was manifest during the history-taking is to be maintained. You look friendly and considerate. You look to see if the patient is comfortable, and if not you adjust his position until he is. You approach the patient knowing that he is undergoing a modified stress test. As Dr. Matthews says, one's approach to the patient who is apprehensive should make it clear that one is aware of his plight, and is determined to set him at ease. If the patient is tense, examination may be difficult and misleading, and proper doctoring, as well as common humanity, demands that he should be as comfortable as is possible in the circumstances.

Some patients do not settle at a first consultation, and blood pressure and heart rate are frequently very much lower on subsequent visits. The occasional patient never gets used to his doctor, even though they get on well, and the consultation is limited to conversation. The only way to obtain a value for the normal resting pulse rate in such patients is to ask them to take it themselves, at home.

A Balanced Approach

Some students, and doctors too, are so worried about getting the signs right that they charge in, head down, like a bull in a china shop. In examining a patient you are perpetrating an assault upon his person which is an impertinence. Obviously, it has got to be done, and in being there the patient is clearly colluding—if often a shade unwillingly—in this assault, but assault it is, especially when the examiner is a student. Your approach will be more balanced if you are determined to get the answer right rather than fearful of getting it wrong.

The Need for Role-Playing

If you are to make the patient feel at ease, which is essential for proper doctoring, you have to school yourself to examine in a way which furthers that objective. If the patient is smelly or has some shocking physical deformity or is extraordinarily attractive or is a very important person indeed, you must proceed as if nothing is unusual. Of course your stance varies from person to person, but you must give the impression that the situation is usual for you, that you have seen every deviation from the norm so many times that it is as routine for you as cleaning your teeth. Of course this is never going to be true, and this is another reason for acting.

Inscrutability

When you discover a sign with a bad prognosis, the look on your face should not reveal your sadness. In *The Journal of a Disappointed Man* the hero, who has multiple sclerosis, observes that when you see a light come into your doctor's eye it does not mean that he has a cure for your condition, but rather that in some way his examination has confirmed his spot diagnosis. He must have seen a series of unskilled doctors; good news, bad news and self-congratulations should only register inwardly. Good news has to be treated like bad news because the patient will detect that then you were pleased, whereas now you are sad. The word "normal" is so pleasing to the ear that I use it frequently during examination: however, one should not say it unless one can disguise its absence.

Unrevealing but Human

The patient watches you all the time for advance information, or for information which you might not reveal at all. You have to ensure that your face does not reveal your findings. Accomplished liars find this easier than those who wear their heart on their sleeve. Some can only achieve security by assuming a cold blandness. This suits some patients, who like a strong silent doctor, and doctors who are ill often choose an icy-mannered colleague to look after them, if they know him to be outstandingly good; the so-called doctor's doctor. If a doctor consults such a colleague he knows that in spite of appearances he is putting himself in safe hands. The ordinary patient has no means of telling that behind the stony exterior there lies a heart of gold. So if you can manage it, without giving the game away, try to look human. Like feeling the spleen, this requires practice. If you believe in absolutely truthful relationships you will by now have decided that this is not the book for you.

Preparation for the Examination of Children

You have to take even more care to reassure children; with adult patients it is best not to talk too much when you are examining them because they know that you cannot concentrate properly if you do. Children on the other hand are reassured by appropriate chatter and questions. Although it distracts you from the job in hand, it distracts them too. They like to try your stethoscope or patellar hammer or torch. They might also like to try your ophthalmoscope, but it may never work again. A supply of sweets may work wonders. Parents, trying to be helpful, may say "The doctor isn't going to hurt you," and this is far from reassuring. Your manner has to convey that the examination is not painful.

GETTING THE HANG OF PHYSICAL SIGNS

Physical signs vary in the ease with which they can be elicited, but none of them is so difficult that the averagely endowed student cannot learn to detect them. Like medical concepts, medical signs are "O" level subjects well within the grasp of anyone who has got into medical school. Their difficulty is analogous to riding a bicycle: anyone who is normal can do it, almost no one can do it first time. Practice makes perfect, and with increasing confidence you can manage it with no hands or with feet on the handlebars. I once saw a circus performer flick six cups and saucers off his foot onto the top of his head while riding a monocycle. The handles of all the cups ended up in the same plane. Finally he flicked a lump of sugar and a spoon into the top cup. It took him seven years to learn to remain stationary on a monocycle and a further seven to learn to catch the cups and saucers. That is about the time it takes to train a doctor, and that level of skill can be achieved with practice and thought.

In the Beginning

It is unlikely that you will approach your first few patients with confidence in your ability to elicit the physical signs. If you do, your confidence is almost certainly misplaced. Rome was not built in a day, and you do have to wait until you have learned to ride that bicycle. When most laymen listen down a stethoscope, for example, they hear nothing at all, unless the murmur is very loud indeed. Medical students hear the heart sounds obscured by borborygmi and breath sounds. You learn to focus out the borborygmi, until you do not actually hear them. I cannot remember when I last heard a bowel sound while listening to the heart. Just as, by selection, you can hear your name mentioned in a conversational tone of voice from the other side of the room at a crowded party, so you must learn the technique of focussing in the things you want to listen to, or feel, while focussing out what is irrelevant. Many years ago I showed a patient to the late Paul Wood, because I thought I could hear a very soft early diastolic murmur, and he confirmed its presence. I then asked him if the patient had a systolic click. He replied that he didn't know because he had been listening to diastole. That was one of the reasons why he was without peer as a diagnostician.

Confidence Limits

Lack of confidence that is soundly based on ignorance is quite different from the determinedly anti-confident attitude which some students adopt. "I can never feel the posterior tibial artery" more or less guarantees that you will never learn how to feel it.

I'm Not Convinced

Another anti-learning device is the "I'm not convinced" reply when "Sir" asks you if you have felt or seen or heard the physical sign he is demonstrating. The word "convinced" makes it sound as if the sign may or may not be there, and that while "Sir" thinks it is, you in the fulness of your experience, disagree. Physical signs, like everything else, have a more or less bell-shaped distribution. Some are so obvious that the patient's spouse can appreciate them. Most are discernible to the average novice after six weeks of training by a skilled teacher. Some are rather difficult and need skilled hands.

A very few signs need virtuoso talents which most people do not possess. Physical signs are appreciated by the special senses, and we are born with a normal distribution of excellences of these systems. One of my colleagues has incredibly good low-frequency auscultatory powers. He can sometimes hear sounds which are inaudible to others, and which we cannot hear even after we have verified their presence on the phonocardiogram. Each physical sign must, by statistical necessity, have its virtuosi, well outside three standard deviations from the normal performance levels. But such performance is necessary for only about one physical sign in a thousand, and while you are learning you should pretend that such signs do not exist at all.

Inventing Signs

What is more common, and is sadly incurable, is the habit of making up physical signs to show your colleagues how clever you are. This pernicious habit, acquired during student days, may still be present on retirement. You should vow never to make up a physical sign, and never to say you see it or feel it or hear it when you don't. Some students say they do because everyone else has, and they don't want to make themselves conspicuous. This is a mistake, and good teachers much prefer it when you speak the truth. They can then take steps to change your technique so that you can elicit the sign, or at any rate to lay a foundation so that you will with more experience. Of course you should not give your teacher the impression that you are saying "I can't feel it, and so it isn't there." The student who challenges the teacher to teach him something, usually remains ignorant. There is no need to grovel; you just put it to "Sir" in a properly therapeutic way. It is the teacher's job to show you how to *elicit* the signs, but the demonstration is no place for debate on the *presence* of the signs.

There are of course some teachers who teach physical signs which are not there. I suppose that they feel that their stock rises if they are seen to be more than normally gifted, and seeing something that no one else can see might just give one some initial kudos. When, however, it turns out to have been a hallucination, much more kudos is lost and the net result is negative. The student is in no position to know whether "Sir" is a liar or not. Such teachers are in a minority, and the word gets round.

The wise teacher acts in entirely the opposite way. When a sign is present but only to the very experienced observer, it is a mistake to demonstrate it to the students. It only serves to lower their confidence, which is what the good teacher should be building up.

Practice Makes Perfect

Having picked your teacher and having decided that he tells the truth, the fruitful attitude is that the onus is entirely on you to acquire the skill to be able to recognise the sign. The teacher shows you the technique of how to elicit a sign, which is almost as important as having the eyes and ears, and then you keep on practising, until you have it by heart. If you find a good example of a sign which you have found difficult, go back and elicit it as often as the patient will willingly let you. Tell the patient what you are doing, because he may be alarmed by your unusual interest in his physical signs.

Dexterity

They say that you begin to make real music only when you know the notes by heart. Physical signs always require concentration, but once you are trained the concentration is on evaluating the signs. During your apprenticeship all your concentration is required merely to elicit them, and you do not make real diagnosis until you have mastered the techniques of examination. Learning to elicit signs is like learning to play the piano. It cannot be done without practice; anyone who is normally gifted and who is properly motivated, can arrive at average professional competence. The patient's confidence increases if he sees that you are eliciting the physical signs dextrously.

Building Your Data Bank

At the beginning of your career, physical signs are moderately difficult to elicit. As you progress, you try to get more out of the sign, and as a result it never becomes so easy to elicit signs that you can do it automatically. The tyro will be able to tell if the tone of a limb is grossly excessive. The expert, at the end of his career, will still have to strive to tell if it is the tiniest bit stiffer than the thousands of normals he has tested. The computer in your head recalls the normal distribution curve of the stiffness of limbs, and tell you whether the limb under examination is outside three standard deviations from the norm or not.

Getting the Best Tools for the Job

It may be true that "A bad workman blames his tools," but good workmen always have good tools. One of the surest ways of acquiring a lifelong inability to elicit a particular sort of physical sign is to "economise" on buying stethoscopes and patellar hammers and ophthalmoscopes. The ophthalmoscope with a light which goes out each time you bend over to examine the fundus is not a bargain, no matter how little you paid for it. Conversely, the best available apparatus is easier to use—that is what you pay extra for—and it puts the onus firmly on your own shoulders. If you are able to say to yourself "Well, I didn't see it, but I never can see anything through my ophthalmoscope," it puts the blame on the ophthalmoscope. If you buy the best one, then you go into action knowing that if the sign is there, your apparatus is capable of transmitting it. The less skilled you are the better the apparatus you need. Most of the apparatus which a doctor needs will last a lifetime, and if it is more expensive than something inferior, you have to remember that the cost is amortised over forty years, and the therapeutic advantage is enormous.

You have to get used to apparatus, and so it is best always to use your own. I find it extremely difficult to use a borrowed stethoscope if it is of a different brand. It takes some days to get used to one which is of equal quality. Some stethoscopes are incapable of transmitting sounds adequately, and similar criticism can be made of most of the few pieces of apparatus which medical students have to buy. Resist the temptation to rush out and buy a stethoscope as an insignia of office as soon as you have passed the preclinical examinations; it may prove to have no other function. Take advice from an expert before you buy.

A tape measure is one of the most valuable instruments you can buy. The value of the observation that one thigh is "slightly wasted" is transformed if you say that it is 40 cm in circumference at a point 18 cm above the patella. The measurements are of value to the next doctor who sees the patient, and allow you to assess the progress of the disease.

The Prejudiced Approach to a Sign

If you suspect, as a result of history-taking and observation of a patient's features, or because of a physical sign you have found, that a patient has a particular disease, you make a tentative diagnosis, and you look for the signs of that condition. You focus your mind on the diagnostic physical sign of that condition, particularly if it is difficult to elicit. You go into action thinking "Where am I likely to make a mistake here?" If, for example, you are not good at auscultation, you ask yourself what the auscultatory physical signs are likely to be if your tentative diagnosis is correct, and you start off looking for those signs, rather than looking at any sign which may be revealed.

Intellectual Honesty

If you use this prejudiced approach, the essential corollary is intellectual honesty. Throughout your career, listen to what people say about physical signs and then make up your own mind about them. No one, no matter how distinguished, should be able to persuade you to say that a sign is present if you cannot elicit it yourself. The fact that you cannot elicit it never means that it is not present, but you should not "find" it simply because someone else does. If you have a strong hunch that you are going to find a particular disease, then look for its diagnostic signs, but never make them up. If they are not there you must abandon, without regret, the spot diagnosis and chase another hare. Man has a dangerous tendency to find what he expects, and you must guard against "findings" which are not there.

Expectant Examination

A familiar phrase in the days before the advent of curative therapy was "expectant therapy." This meant that you waited for symptoms to develop and then gave something to suppress or abolish them. In physical examination you should maintain an expectant attitude. You have your preconceived notion, but in the course of examining the patient for the signs of that condition your mind is at the same time kept open, so that any other physical sign which presents is allowed to exert its full weight on the diagnosis. As you proceed, the diagnosis may have to change several times, but it gets nearer to the truth each time.

Slightly Pregnant

Physical signs are either there, not there, or there but you cannot elicit them. Many, like bronchospasm or the jugular venous pressure or the intensity of murmurs, can vary from minute to minute, may "disappear" and may then return. Physical signs of diseases which develop and then wane have a bell-shaped intensity course. Take for example jaundice. This correlates in intensity with the level of bilirubin in the blood. There is always some bilirubin in the blood. Either we make allowance for that, or it has such a small effect on the overall colour of the skin that everyone would agree that there was no jaundice. As, say, the infective hepatitis runs its course, the intensity of the jaundice will first become evident to those who have good colour discrimination and colour memory (absolute pitch for colour) and to those who look carefully, then become obvious to all, and finally wane, becoming gradually less obvious with the passage of time. Changes in such physical signs are often the most sensitive indicator of a change in the patient's condition.

Physical signs such as jaundice and cyanosis and the character of the pulse which are always present in the normal person and are merely accentuated by disease are more difficult than, say, a murmur, which is either present or absent.

Students are encouraged not to sit on the fence and this is good training because you have to commit yourself. Teachers bristle if students say that the patient is "slightly" jaundiced: "Either you think he is jaundiced or you don't." But in fact, as everything has to start somewhere, the degree of jaundice may be low enough to make two skilled observers disagree as to whether it is present or not. The only response which a proper doctor can have to a physical sign is to try and elicit it, and then to make up his mind whether it is present or not. It is perfectly reasonable to say "Yes, the patient is jaundiced, but the degree of jaundice is very slight." It is also perfectly proper to say "I think the patient is jaundiced, but the degree of jaundice is so slight that I might be making a mistake."

The Observer Error Error

Doctors vary in their skill, and in their honesty too, and in unskilled circles a great deal of fuss is made about the presence or absence of physical signs. In skilled circles disagreement is rare and is confined to those signs which are of such low intensity that they could be confused by a skilled observer with normality.

If a skilled neurologist elicits an extensor plantar response, and a skilled ear, nose and throat surgeon, examining at the same time, considers it to be flexor, that is not observer error, that is a mistake. The fact that a man is medically qualified certainly does not mean that he is still competent to elicit all physical signs, and this supposition is the basis of the incredible literature on observer error. Most people who are skilled are engaged in healing the sick and their minds are directed to the problems this raises. They are usually busy, and uninterested in quantifying how wrong the unskilled can be on the subject of physical signs, so they are unwilling to participate in trials of observer error. However, the doctor who usually gets the signs wrong is much more interested in showing that no one else gets them right either, so he gathers the butcher, the baker and the odd epidemiologist and shows that none of them agrees with each other, nor do they agree with the findings of the good-natured specialist who has been brow-beaten into participating in the trial.

The news that no two observers can agree about the presence or absence of a particular sign percolates down to the students, who feel that if no one can agree about signs there is little point in trying to learn how to detect them. In fact, in skilled circles, the disagreement is limited to marginal cases. It is also true that this level of skill can be achieved in months rather than years. There is such a thing as observer error, but the term does not mean disagreement between unskilled observers. Teaching should be confined to physical signs which are unequivocal, and the student should regard each physical sign which is demonstrated without scepticism. If you are wondering whether the sign is there or not, you are unlikely to elicit it.

The Seminar Approach

In preclinical years the student is encouraged to give his opinion on papers and on what he is taught. The seminar approach, in which all views are taken as being equal, prevails, and I am not in a position to say whether this approach is the best one in that period. In clinical teaching it is not. Whereas the student's view on the comprehensibility of his teachers is important, his view of the content of what he is taught is rarely of interest. Expertise in physical signs flows down the concentration gradient; the student has but to remain fully permeable and learning will inevitably follow. Signs are the bricks and mortar of diagnosis, and successful treatment depends largely on the ability to elicit them.

Tests Cannot Replace Signs

The development of special tests which are thought to give a more reliable answer than the observer-error-riddled physical signs has contributed to students' lack of interest in these signs. Most tests are expensive, time-consuming and not without dangers. Generally, they can only be fully interpreted in the context of the symptoms and signs. Tests are of course essential, and will be discussed fully in Chapter 5, but they are full of pitfalls; complete diagnosis cannot usually be made without the history, the examination and the special tests.

Primum non nocere

Throughout the examination you should be aware of the effect which your examination of the patient is having on him. The physical sign which most interests you, and which you show to your friends, may be unconnected with the patient's condition. If you are taking the opportunity of familiarising yourself with the normal fundus occuli, you may spend a good deal of time looking at it and discussing it. Even if the patient has normal vision and has presented with indigestion, he may well conclude that you have found something wrong with his eyes. Introduce your friend with "Do you mind if I show my friend a normal eye?"

If you ask your teacher "Is that a flexor response?" the patient's anxiety may increase, because he will not know that this is a normal finding. If instead you ask "Is that a normal plantar response?" the teacher can say "Yes, it is." If it is not, the teacher can say whatever he thinks is suitable. Sometimes students and doctors who behave impeccably during the history-taking seem to forget that the patient is conscious during examination. Questions, or answers, which make the patient think, rightly or wrongly, that he has some abnormality, must be avoided. Keep a careful guard on your tongue. Whenever possible, wait until the patient is out of earshot before asking any questions which may have sinister overtones. You must remember that your threshold for anxiety-producing words is much higher than the patient's. Words like "heart failure" may only mean the occasional diuretic to you, but to the patient they sound like a death sentence. Words like heart block or tumour are particularly unfortunate because they sound dreadful although they are often innocuous. Remember too that you are more likely than not to have got it all wrong, and your ignorance must not be allowed to upset the patient. You know that what you say is evidence of your ignorance, but the patient cannot know that.

It has become fashionable now to mock circumlocutions. "As we doctors call it" has become a joke. The modern, sophisticated patient is said to have learned what the long words mean. In fact the majority of patients is not well informed, and words like hepatomegaly are outside most people's comprehension, whereas "a large liver" is inside everybody's vocabulary. If you think that the patient might understand and be upset, err on the safe side and say nothing. There is always tomorrow. In proper doctoring, treatment of the whole patient has priority over everything else.

THE ACTUAL EXAMINATION

Many patients are unrelaxed because they are under stress, and your manner during the history-taking will have been directed towards making the patient relax so that you can examine him properly, in order to come to the right diagnosis. Your manner builds up the patient's confidence in you so that ultimately he will be pleased to take your advice. Immaculate history-taking techniques must be followed by immaculate examination techniques, based on respect for the patient's body and mind.

The Demeanour of the Patient

Throughout the history-taking and the examination you scrutinise the patient for subtle diagnostic clues which reveal the effect that his illness is having on him. You observe the way in which he carries out ordinary tasks when he thinks that he is unobserved. His gait, the way he gets up from a chair, the way he picks things up or carries his belongings, may reveal abnormalities which he may be able to control when he is performing special tests for you. As Feinstein says, "The evidence includes such items as the expression on the face, the sweat on the brow, the coherence of a statement and the vigour of a gesture."

You watch the patient to see if his behaviour fits with the symptoms he reports or with the disease with which he has been labelled. The patient who strides over to the examination couch and swings himself onto it with agility is unlikely to have peritonitis.

Laying Hands on the Patient

Your clean hands must be warm and dry. If they are not, wash them and dry them thoroughly. If washing facilities are not available, dry your hands and warm them by rubbing them together. It is interesting to watch the patient's face as you do this; it tells you that the experience is unusual for him. If your hands are still cold, you can warm up by gripping the patient's forearm, having forewarned him of what you are about to do. Always warm your stethoscope before use by holding the chestpiece in your closed fist and rubbing it briskly. If you are wearing the stethoscope, make sure it is "switched off" because the noise is deafening and impairs auscultation.

Dr. Matthews tells the story of a group of prisoners of war in Japanese hands who were liberated by the Russians. The Russians decided to execute the Japanese guards, but first asked the prisoners if anyone should be spared. The prisoners asked that the Japanese doctor should be let off, because he always warmed his hands before examining them. Warming your hands could be life saving.

First Physical Contact

Generally the only other experience the patient will have of being touched is the "loving" situation, and then usually only by "lovers" or by parents. The doctor is not in either of these positions, and before you put a hand on the patient you have to look him in the eye in order to convey that you are aware of his thoughts and feelings, and that he can rely on you to infringe his dignity as little as possible, while relentlessly pursuing the diagnosis with a view to treatment. To the uninitiated this may seem a tall order for a single look, but you are more than halfway there if you smile warmly and reassuringly. The rest follows when you gain in confidence.

Examination starts with sight and smell. Some diseases and drugs have characteristic smells, and one is most likely to notice them as you first enter the examination cubicle, or as you approach the patient.

The first physical contact with a patient, often feeling the pulse, is an important moment. The patient can tell a lot from the way you handle his flesh. Firstly it must be handled with respect. Even if it is dirty you must pick it up in a professional manner. The amount of force which is required to elicit the various physical signs varies from a light touch to firm, and you have to use enough force to enable you to elicit the sign. If the patient has some condition which is painful, even the lightest touch may be exquisitely painful. I remember one of my teachers telling us that if one knocked the bedframe with one's knee, the patient with gout would wince with pain, and that one could tell in this way if he was better. When all twelve of my fellow students had thus tested the patient I realised the price patients have to pay for student education.

Forewarn the Patient

In one way or another, the patient should be aware of what you are going to do. If it is something unexceptional, such as feeling his pulse, then making your way, at a steady pace, with obvious intent is enough. If you want to do a rectal examination, which is more of an assault, then you ask/say what you are about to do. It would be silly to make such a fuss in asking permission that you made the patient anxious or indeed made him refuse his permission. If you say "I would like to examine your rectum"—or "back passage" if you think that he may not understand—in a tone which implies that it has to be done but that you are asking his permission, then his dignity is preserved. If the patient is forewarned he will not be taken by surprise; he may not have expected, or may not see the need for, the examination which you are about to do and an unexpected assault is a shock.

How Would I Feel?

Throughout your career you should ask yourself whether, if you were the same age and as ill and as frail as the patient, you would submit to the assault which you propose. If the answer is yes, go ahead; if it is no, forego, gracefully, the assault. Do not console yourself with the view—once widely held, now fortunately dying, but not as quickly as it should—that "patients are different." They aren't; students are embryo patients, and there is no correlation between education or social class and sensitivity.

The Threshold of Discomfort

Both patients and doctors are normally distributed for sensitivity to pain. One hopes that the doctor's curve of sensibility to the pain he is causing is well over to the "good" side of normal, but it has to be said that some doctors are rough with patients. Minimal roughness compatible with eliciting the sign is the aim. If you are so gentle that you can never feel the spleen, then you are too gentle. Do not ask yourself whether you are gentle or not, because the answer is bound to be that you are. Ask yourself each time you elicit a sign whether you could have done it with less pressure. Ask yourself what information will be gained from handling, and whether it will affect treatment.

The tenser the patient is, the more sensitive he is to discomfort. Rough or unsympathetic handling makes him tense. From the practical point of view alone, the tense patient is more difficult to examine. Tension makes the cardiovascular system abnormal, and makes examination of the abdomen and of the central nervous system much more difficult.

The Uncontorted Clinician

As with the par golf swing, for feeling the spleen, your feet must be in the right position. You have to be facing in the appropriate direction, so that you do not have to twist your arm or your wrists, because the feeling of discomfort from the wrist distracts part of the mind from feeling the spleen. You should examine for each physical sign from the "best" position for yourself, each time. I am unable to hear as well when I auscultate while standing on the patient's left side, as may be necessary when examining patients in their homes. If you are extremely tall or short, or suffer some physical disability, you may have to invent your own positions to circumvent these handicaps.

Positioning the Patient

In order to allow you to concentrate your whole mind on the estimation of the sign in question, and to extract the maximum of information from it, the patient must not only be comfortable and relaxed, but also lying in the position which makes it easiest for you to elicit the sign. You must put, and maintain, the patient in that position.

Patients may "help" the doctor. Most patients turn their head away when you are looking at their neck veins, and this tension of the skin makes the veins very difficult to see. Others hold their breath when you are listening to the front of their chest because they do not want to breathe on your face, but if you are listening to the breath sounds, or to the effect of breathing on heart sounds, this is counterproductive. If you say "breath normally" many patients respond with an abnormal "saw-toothed" pattern of breathing, and it is best to wait until they are forced to take a breath. In fact the larger than usual breath that they take in these circumstances is often helpful in determining whether or not the second heart sound splits normally with respiration.

A patient will be unable to relax if he is trying to work out what he ought to be doing, so you must show from the outset that you will put his limbs exactly where you want them, and that all he has to do is to leave them limp. If you say "Let me feel your pulse," the patient will raise his arm. It is better, for the distant objective of eliciting his abdominal reflexes, if you take up the arm yourself, hold it firmly, and put it back when you have finished. If you do this from the start the patient gets to understand that you will put him where you want him, and that you will not drop him. He can relax.

It is often forgotten that patients have backs, which repay examination. If you want a patient to sit up you have to have his help unless he is too ill to assist. There is no harm in helping everyone up, however, as it perpetuates the feeling that you are controlling the movements.

The Order of Examination

If you examine patients well, their tension diminishes as the examination continues. Thus, if you keep the most important part of the examination until the end, you may get a truer blood pressure reading, or a better examination of the central nervous system, or a more relaxed abdomen. Patients expect you to examine the system at fault first, and the earlier you make the diagnosis, the sooner you can concentrate on its finer points. But in the tense patient it pays to look at that system again when they have settled. If you wish to examine something when it is in a state of maximum relaxation, do it before you make the patient sit up to examine his back, because the sitting up disturbs the relaxation.

The Mental Check-list Approach

Examination should be carried out with teutonic thoroughness. As far as possible you should do the same tests in the same order on everyone. In this way you establish an automatic routine for the order of examination and are less likely to forget anything—although of course the examination itself must never be automatic. You may have some procedures—palpation of the breasts and rectal examination are two examples—which you may decide to perform on all patients as a routine. You tack them onto your examinations at an appropriate moment, so that these too become semi-automatic. If the patient is too ill for a full examination or if there is not enough time, you note down carefully what you have found, taking particular care to note everything which in future days—or even years—it may be important to know about. You also leave a space for description at a later date of those systems which you were unable to examine at the first consultation.

Opportunism in Examination

There are, however, exceptions to the rule of always following the same order of examination. For example, in infants or in the very sick, if they happen to be lying on one side or prone, you take the opportunity to examine the presenting part. This saves moving the patient, and a sleeping child may offer a not-to-be-repeated opportunity for examination. If the left ear presents, examine it first. It may not present again. With crying children, you seize on a gap between cries to auscultate or to feel the abdomen or to examine the most important part. In infants you may be able to do this while they are sleeping or drowsy after a feed.

Failed Physical Examination

Once you are trained, the commonest cause of failure to elicit signs is carelessness. If you forget to look for a sign, you will not find it. If you look for it in a slapdash way, you are likely to get it wrong. Such lapses are intolerable in professional men and women. If you do your best but miss a sign, that is perfectly acceptable, but if you cannot be bothered to do the job properly, your licence to practise should be withdrawn.

EVALUATING THE PHYSICAL SIGNS

There are many books which tell you about physical signs; I intend only to give a general approach to eliciting them.

The term physical sign covers both normal and abnormal findings. The fact that a patient has not got exophthalmos is as noteworthy as its presence. When you detect a physical sign you evaluate its features, so that you could paint a picture of it. You estimate the degree of the sign, deciding whether it is slight, moderate, severe or gross—or in shorthand grades 1 to 4. As there is no official grading method it is as well to write this down as 1/4, 2/4, 3/4 and 4/4, as this allows other people too to assess changes in the sign over days or years. Some phenomena are all or none, and are not susceptible to grading, but there are surprisingly few of them. Even a fractured femur can be "badly" or "not so badly" broken, and the badness can be graded. Grade 1 indicates only just discernible and grade 4 means fully developed, and the two intervening grades lie in between.

Physical signs are not just "items" to be elicited. They are the physical signs of the underlying pathophysiology. As an example, you feel the pulse not for itself but because it is a non-invasive method of estimating haemodynamics, and as you feel it you ask yourself what it is telling you about the performance of the heart.

The Inquisitional Approach

With each sign, you put it to yourself that it is either more so than normal, or less so than normal, or normal. You examine each hypothesis in turn. You say to yourself "Well, it certainly isn't less than normal." Then you add "It could be normal, or more than normal." Having eliminated less than normal, you have one more try at less than normal, in order to make certain that you have not eliminated it prematurely. If you are certain that it is not less than normal, you go over the same ground again with normal and greater than normal. "Why isn't it normal?," you ask yourself. "Well, it's really too much for normal," you reply. "If I was presented with this sign without any previous knowledge about the patient, would it still seem more than normal?"

You subject each sign to this inquisition, and what you are doing is comparing it with your visual or auditory or palpatory image of all the normal and all the abnormal examples of that sign which you have ever examined. In addition to flicking through your memory file, you have to make adjustments for age or sex or excitement or pain or the ambient temperature or obesity or deformity or any other factor which will itself modify the sign in the absence of actual disease. You may be able to use the patient "as his own control." If he has pain in his left ankle you look for differences between it and his right ankle, and this process can be applied to abdominal "guarding" or even to murmurs. If you are not sure whether a sound you are hearing is a soft diastolic rumble or external noise, you can listen in the same position on the other side of the chest.

To each characteristic of the sign you apply the same inquisitional, comparative technique. "Does it go up to the second sound?" or "Is there a notch on it?" or "Does it pulsate or is the pulsation transmitted?" Each aspect has to be considered and compared, so that in the end you know all about the sign.

It is evident that you need as much experience of normal and abnormal examination as you can possibly get. You need constant practice in order to keep your sign-eliciting powers in tip-top condition. The slightest deviation from the norm may be important. After a fortnight's holiday, it takes a day or two before your ability to detect signs returns to peak level.

The Signs Must Be Compatible with Each Other

All aspects of the sign must be mutually compatible. If they are not, you have to re-estimate the sign. To some extent signs can be used to check on each other. If you see an "a" wave in the neck, it is inconsistent with a diagnosis of atrial fibrillation. So if you have "found" both signs, one of them must be wrong. You go back to the neck and make sure that it really is an "a" wave, and this time an added aspect of your inquisition is your new knowledge about the "fibrillation." One or other sign is wrong, or more accurately you have been mistaken about one of them. Without observer bias, whilst being entirely biased in favour of getting the answer right, you re-examine both signs dispassionately. You do not say to yourself "He is in atrial fibrillation so it cannot be an 'a' wave," but you see if you still think it is an "a" wave now that you think that he is in fibrillation. The venous wave either precedes, is synchronous with, or follows the carotid pulse. Examine each hypothesis in turn. If you still think it is an "a" wave and you simply cannot bring yourself to call it anything else, you re-examine the auscultatory sign, and feel the pulse again.

There are no rules in physical examination which forbid you to re-examine when you are in doubt; there are no proscriptions against changing the patient's position, or exercising him. You may move to where the light is better, or to where it is cooler or warmer or quieter; you may do anything within reason which facilitates the evaluation of the signs. If after this sort of examination the signs are still incompatible, you seek a second opinion, or do a test, if one is available, which will resolve the difficulty. There are many situations where there is no test, and there are other situations where the test shows that your interpretation of a sign is wrong.

When the Facts Don't Fit

Occasionally, even when you know the diagnosis, you are still certain that your interpretation of the sign was correct, and this belief may be shared by all the other trained observers. Even when you know the diagnosis for certain, you are unable to take any other view of this incompatible physical sign. This awkward aspect of physical signs is a trial to the beginner, but it is stimulating to the experienced. You approach a diagnosis which you have got wrong before in the knowledge that you might be getting it wrong again, and this is stimulating. After years of experience the total of occasions where the signs do not fit the diagnosis becomes substantial, and this keeps you on the *qui vive* and prevents complacency. Although it is infuriating to be beaten by a physical sign, I always take pleasure in the reconfirmation that medicine is an art as well as a science.

Forme fruste

Quite often, particularly in general medicine, there are not enough signs to permit you to make a diagnosis. Teachers prefer to demonstrate patients who have signs, and whose signs fit, so "atypical" patients are less likely to be taught on, but you will come across them later. The incidence of patients with signs which do not fit is low, and the student should not take refuge in the inexacting philosophy that they often do not fit. For practical purposes, if the signs do not fit it is because you have got one or more of them wrong. This should condition your approach until you become an expert at physical signs; until that time, if the signs do not fit you should re-examine the patient.

Never miss an opportunity to re-examine a patient. Once you have done it, look up the notes and see what you wrote down last time. This check on your "repeatability" is an invaluable learning technique and, once you have learned, ensures that your standards are maintained.

Keeping an Open Mind

During the history-taking you are making your symptomatic diagnosis. During the examination you are refining your symptomatic diagnosis by the addition of the examination diagnosis. The ultimate diagnosis may be changed from either of these earlier diagnoses by tests. The passage of time often makes diagnosis clearer even if nothing changes except the stress which you lay on some aspect. Your mind must be kept open to change when the earlier diagnosis becomes untenable. For this reason, and because diagnosis carries more weight after the process is complete, it is a mistake to tell the patient your diagnosis before you have reached the final one. Sometimes patients, in their anxiety to know whether they are abnormal or not, will ask you in the middle of an examination. I always ask them to wait until I have got to the end, even when I am "certain" that they are normal. It prolongs their agony of unknowing, but the reassurance is more reassuring if it comes after a complete examination, and a good deal of damage is done if you find that some later evidence forces you to recant your premature reassurance.

4. IN THE WARD

THE PRACTICE of medicine in the ward differs in a number of ways from outpatient medicine. The first difference is the tempo. Outpatient medicine is more difficult and challenging because you have to make quick decisions, on less evidence, and without the assistance of the junior medical and nursing staff; on the other hand, as so many patients are normal, many are not seriously ill, and others although ill can be easily treated, the average amount of time spent on each patient is shorter. That is not to say that reassurance of a healthy but worried person is less valuable or difficult or time-consuming than the treatment of pneumonia, but in general the pace is faster. Ward patients are talked to and examined at greater length, and they are subjected to investigations which require explanation, evaluation and consultation.

THE EFFECT OF WARD LIFE ON THE PATIENT

Although ex-servicemen, public schoolboys and ex-prisoners will have experienced communal living, most people find that admission to a ward takes a good deal of getting used to. Even if you have never sat on a bed pan, screened visually but not acoustically from an interested audience of twenty or thirty people, you can readily imagine that the experience might be costive.

In outpatients the patient is, as already described, not his usual self. Once admitted, he becomes even less so. In outpatients he knows that no major procedure will be carried out on the spot. Furthermore, he knows that the ordeal is to be short-lived, and that after an hour or two he will be back in the "real" world again, where he feels at home, and has a busy life to lead. In the ward, in sharp contrast, his time commitment is open-ended and the job, appointments, hobbies, duties and family ties which established his place in the world are abruptly suspended. He has nothing to do, and all his badges of office in society are removed. This is one reason why visiting time is so important for patients; visits from friends and relations serve to re-establish the patient's identity, and undo the harm done to his ego by admission to the ward. The fact that he has had to be admitted augments his outpatient fears of the disease, and for his future. The admission itself may have given rise to anxieties about his work or his home circumstances. If the patient is unintelligent or unreasonable the burden of disease may be even more upsetting for him.

Being Nice to Inpatients

Ward staff, from Sister down to the merest crossing sweeper, all reinforce the patient's "anomie" if they are anything less than exceptionally considerate. Ordinary consideration is not enough, because the patient in the ward often behaves in a manner which is quite unlike his own, and which is frequently hypersensitive and silly. Sensible people become obsessed with the idea that Sister prefers the patient in the next bed, or that the ward maid is giving them smaller portions of food, or that the doctors are giving more attention to the man opposite. Very often the man opposite gets more attention because his condition demands it, but this does not prevent the patient who is steadily getting better with minimal attention, from being jealous.

Ward staff, including students, have to take care not to reinforce any irrational feelings that the patient may have. The doctor's manner should be as considerate as it would be when talking to someone who had been terrified by some awful event, or overwhelmed by bereavement.

If you recognise that admission to hospital makes people behave abnormally, you will be able to take up a professional attitude to their behaviour. An inexplicable outburst of rage or of crying can be looked upon as a "toxic" manifestation of the disease, rather than as bloody-mindedness. If you cannot suffer fools gladly, you should take up laboratory work. The proper doctor maintains his equanimity at all times. A patient once told Geoffrey Evans that he wasn't getting anything to eat. Instead of telling him not to be a damned fool, Evans rounded on Sister and said "Are you starving this man?" The patient, recognising a just man when he saw one, was won over and agreed to accept the food which he had been refusing. Variations on this sort of response are constantly required from a proper doctor, and from a proper Sister too.

The Advantages of Being Admitted to the Ward

Over and above the necessity for admitting patients, there are advantages which come from the same sources as the harmful effects. Most patients adapt to being admitted, and when the stress of outside life is removed they may come to terms with their disease and its implications for the first time. After "institutionalisation" has occurred they are prepared to accept advice which they would not have taken in outpatients.

TALKING TO PATIENTS

The ward patient has all the time in the world to talk, and the doctor should adjust his speed to that, wherever possible. A brisk ward round with a huge retinue, dashing from bed to bed, may be all that is required for the patient's physical welfare, but it does not treat the whole patient. A round on your own, or with the houseman, or a nurse, taken at an unhurried pace is therapeutic in itself.

Ward Sisters used to frown when a doctor sat on a patient's bed because it rumpled the sheets, but it has now become acceptable to do so. It makes the patient feel that you are not going to rush off and it gives him an opportunity to ask a question to which he had previously assumed you were too busy to answer. This concept of the busy doctor is firmly embedded in patients' minds and you have to disabuse them of it; answering questions is an integral part of proper doctoring. If you feel that the patient has a question which he does not raise even when the two of you are alone, you can often answer it unasked. Many of the questions which trouble people with particular diseases are foreseeable, and you learn others with experience.

When talking to a patient who is in bed, stand near the head of the bed. Do not stand at the foot of the bed and shout. You should lower your voice—other patients will be listening in, and the patient has the right to privacy. The feeling of privacy is enhanced if you close the curtains round the bed.

Although patients spend a good deal of time telling each other what the doctor said and discussing and comparing their situations, in the first instance this information is confidential, and the patient must have the right to filter out those parts of it which he feels are unsuitable for broadcasting. The doctor can have no idea which parts will be considered unsuitable, and must treat it all as though it is to go no further. A small side-room off the ward, where conversations with patients and their relatives can be held in private, is a boon. Patients may ask you about a fellow patient if they are worried about him. Without giving offence, you must give non-committal or non-revealing answers.

Talking Directly to the Patient

During ward rounds it is often necessary to ask Sister or one of the doctors about some technical aspect of the patient's disease; but questions about the patient's symptoms should be directed to the patient. If you say "Is he walking better, Sister?," it makes it clear that in your view the patient is not sufficiently reliable to be able to give an opinion. Of course many patients are not reliable, but you ask them directly because it is insulting if you don't. If Sister disagrees with the patient's estimate of his progress she can either say so at the time, and then all three of you can discuss the matter, or if she thinks that would be unhelpful, she can tell you her opinion later.

Over the Patient's Head

The patient lies there, a yard or so below one's line of vision, and there may be a tendency to forget about him. It is perfectly legitimate to discuss aspects of his disease in his presence, and many patients like it because it gives them an opportunity to learn about their disease. But though he is out of sight, he must not be out of mind, and everything which is said in his presence must be censored. I once heard a consultant on a ward round ask his registrar "What's his survival time?"; the reply came back "Ten days." The patient needed a good deal of convincing that they were referring to the fate of some labelled red cells. If there is any chance that the patient may be alarmed, the remark should not be made. If it is made, the doctor should make it clear that the remark did not apply in his particular case. If said convincingly this may be accepted, but it is better not to make such remarks. The ward round is essentially a series of consultations with individual patients, and all other personnel are in subsidiary roles. The patient holds the centre of the stage, and although he understands that you have to discuss him with other people he is the star of the show.

"My Student Says . . ."

A medical student may make friends with a patient, and spend a lot of time talking to him. Patients are often fishing for information about their disease and students should remember that they are not in charge of the patient, nor are they knowledgeable enough either of disease or of human nature, to tell the patients anything. At the slightest sign that the conversation has moved into personal medical channels, the student should say that he doesn't really know enough about the situation to talk about it, and that anything he said might be wrong and misleading. The student loses face, but that is infinitely preferable to damaging the patient. Students are not qualified to give advice until they are registered, and even then they have to make sure that what they say is in line with the intentions of whoever has overall responsibility for the patient. This applies not only to students but to all who come into contact with the patient.

DECISION-MAKING AT THE BEDSIDE

One characteristic of a good clinician is his ability to make the "right" decision in evenly balanced situations. Whilst he may reasonably take pride in this accomplishment, the patient derives comfort from the concept that in his case, the decision is cut and dried. A surgeon I worked for was wont to discuss the site of the incision at the bedside. When he and his aides had marked the alternatives with the nail of their index finger, the triple responses on the patient's abdomen looked like a plan for a complicated motorway junction. The patient's face revealed his alarm. Even a discussion about whether a patient is fit enough for convalescence raises a question of premature discharge in the patient's mind. The patient wants to hear that he is now ready for convalescence or that he will be ready by a certain date, or that it is too early to say when he will be ready. Whenever it is, he wants to leave the hospital confident that the time is exactly ripe.

Discussion about management should take place outside the ward, where doubts about the wisdom of a course of action can be debated in full. Some clinicians walk out of earshot and discuss the patient, but they may be within the range of another patient who may well retail a garbled version of what was said. Although the patient is out of earshot, he may be able to see the facial expressions and gestures of his medical advisers, and will draw his own conclusions. A kindly physician I worked for would say to the patient "We are now going to the other end of the ward to discuss your case," which I felt provoked anxiety. If the decision is difficult, and further discussion is required which might upset the patient, an acceptable strategy is to tell the patient that you are thinking about his problem and will come to a decision later. Patients are pleased to think that their fate is decided by weighing up. It is tossing up which alarms them.

THE MEGAROUND

Generally, ward rounds are conducted with the personnel who are directly involved in the treatment of the patient, and these small rounds are the most satisfactory from all points of view. Sometimes for teaching purposes, or for the demonstration of unusual or interesting or difficult problems, a large crowd descends upon the ward. Patients should be told that a large round is about to visit, and all patients who are to be examined or taught on should be forewarned, and their permission and cooperation obtained. The number of people who examine the patient should be restricted to that number which the patient seems happy to allow. Examinations should cease well before he shows overt signs of satiety.

In the excitement of discussion on a large round, there is a tendency to forget that the patient is present. Nothing which is said should be antitherapeutic. Bored participants on the fringes of these large rounds should behave in a professional manner. Although you may be out of sight of your chief or of the patient, other patients will be observing your behaviour pattern.

DODGING THE COLUMN

As a registrar I had a useful lesson from a ward Sister. One of our patients was dying and I found the strain of daily visits with, as I thought, nothing to offer, discomfiting, embarrassing and emotionally upsetting because the patient was a nice woman whose illness had been long drawn out and unpleasant. As I approached the bed, I seized on the fact that her eyes were closed to tell Sister that I would not disturb her as she was "resting." "Oh yes you will, doctor" said Sister, and she told me that it was essential to maintain interest, that the visit itself was therapeutic, and that there was almost always some aspect of the patient's condition which would justify an encouraging remark. If not, juggling with the drugs would convince the patient that she was not being abandoned as hopeless. When you cannot cure, you are still bound to do whatever you can.

CHANGING THE MEDICATION

Many patients who are admitted to the wards will have been on long-term medication. A common sequel of admittance is that all the medicines which the patient brings with him are stopped and new ones substituted. If the patient has been admitted because his long-term medication was unsatisfactory, this may be the correct thing to do, but frequently the patient is admitted for some other reason, or the dosage of medicaments simply needs adjusting, in which case a changeover to new drugs may be disadvantageous to the patient because it takes time to get the dosage right, and new drugs mean new side effects. Frequently the drugs will be stopped by a newly qualified houseman, and he may be undoing months of work by someone who is more experienced. The merit of each drug should be assessed on the basis of its effectiveness in that particular patient, and on its suitability in the circumstance of this particular admission to the ward. If the admitting doctor is unfamiliar with the drug, he should look it up before he stops it. If he is unfamiliar with it and the dosage needs adjusting, he may prefer to change to another drug which he has experience of using. There is no doubt that you get better results with drugs if you have experience of handling them. But this improvement is "bought" at the expense to the patient of a period of experimentation. The patient's faith in the doctor who prescribed the drugs is impaired if they are all stopped, and they should only be stopped when they are clearly inferior to some newer drug. I have heard housemen explaining at the bedside that the patient's previous medication was hopelessly inadequate, and such statements, whether correct or not, are antitherapeutic.

DISCHARGE FROM HOSPITAL

Discharge is a crucial event for the patient. Each patient should be privately interviewed by the registrar who has supervised the admission. The patient should be given a summary of his situation and the opportunity grasped to ensure that he understands what he has been told on previous occasions. Clear instructions about management of his illness should be given, and the patient must be allowed enough time to ask questions or to register any complaints. An appointment should be arranged for a follow-up visit to outpatients, unless this is unnecessary.

If the patient is to continue to take drugs after discharge from hospital, he should be given an adequate supply to tide him over until his general practitioner can see him; if the dosage is likely to need adjustment in the altered circumstances of life outside hospital, he should be told of the possibility, forewarned about the symptoms and signs of inappropriate dosage, and told what action he should take.

Putting the General Practitioner in the Picture

The general practitioner depends on the hospital for an adequate account of the patient's stay in hospital. The findings, the decisions which were made, the therapy administered, and when necessary to be continued, should be described in enough detail to enable the practitioner to take up the reins again smoothly.

Discharge summaries frequently arrive too late, and every effort should be made to get them out in time for the practitioner to read them before he sees the patient again. When this is not possible, the patient should be given a note with the basic information which the practitioner needs, especially the dosage of drugs. The patient should feel that the hospital and the practitioner are both part of one integrated service.

"Can I Go Home?"

Another example of the "insanity" of inpatients, which will not seem quite so insane if you have been an inpatient yourself, is their preoccupation with getting out of the hospital regardless of whether or not this will damage their health. Doctor patients, who often, but not invariably, realise the consequences of such premature discharge, may behave in the same way. The boredom, the noise, the discipline, the food, the lack of privacy, and the depression which results from being surrounded by other sick people, combine with the effects of disease and its treatment to make people ignore their instinct for self-preservation in their desire to escape. On a ward round a student told William Evans that the patient they were examining wished to take his own discharge. "Why do you think he wants to do that?"

asked Evans. "I've no idea sir," the student replied, "we have hardly begun his treatment." Evans turned to the registrar and said "Make certain that this student is warded before he qualifies."

Patients Who Take Their Own Discharge

Patients who discharge themselves rarely come to any harm, and doctors who advise against it tend to err on the "safe" side, as of course they should. When faced with a patient who has summoned up the courage to take his own discharge, against everyone's advice, having signed all those forms, remember that he has had a great deal to put up with, and that he may not have the self-discipline to continue. He may also have motives for discharge which he is unwilling to reveal. Remember too, that you may behave in exactly the same way in similar circumstances. Your natural exasperation at the thought that all the good work may be undone, to say nothing of the annoyance at having your advice rejected "after all you have done," should be concealed. You are paid to treat the whole patient, and it is he who has to suffer the treatment. Practising medicine is its own reward, and the patients owe neither compliance nor gratitude. It is your duty to make it perfectly clear to the patient if you feel that he should remain in hospital. Your manner must be neither hectoring nor disapproving nor threatening. It should be doctorly; if complications develop because the patient leaves prematurely, you are prepared to treat them. The patient has not "blotted his copy book," and no offence has been taken.

WARD NOTES

When the patient is in the ward there may be no necessity to make notes of changes in his condition or of the treatment policy, because these matters are very much in people's minds, and the staff may be too busy to write them down. When, at a later date, an attempt is made to ascertain the course of events during the admission, the notes usually prove inadequate. Students and junior doctors can do much to remedy this situation by making a précis of the important events and policy changes.

5. INVESTIGATION

IF THERE were no risks or disadvantages, all relevant tests would be done on all patients, and for a "complete check up" many irrelevant tests would be done too. Tests are time-consuming and expensive, and if they are clearly unnecessary, doing them increases the waiting time for patients who really need the test, besides wasting scarce resources. Even the simplest test can be dangerous; there have been exceptional reports of gangrene following venepuncture. The amount of discomfort and danger varies from test to test; some carry a morbidity even in the best hands, which makes the "price" that the patient has to pay for information quite substantial. What is less commonly acknowledged is that in the worst hands—and it is a statistical inevitability that some of us must have them—the morbidity is considerably higher, and the quality of the information which is obtained may be low. This alters the "price."

FACTORS INFLUENCING THE ORDERING OF TESTS

Reassuring the Patient

Some patients are made anxious by tests, and approximately an equal number are relieved by them, or are relieved by knowing that the test has proved to be normal. The doctor must judge which type of patient he is dealing with. Some patients are determined to have a certain test and will not be satisfied until it is done. If the test they wish to have and do not need is risky, then they must remain unsatisfied, but if it is safe it may be therapeutic to do it.

Screening Tests

There is a school of thought which does all the tests—or at least all those which are relatively safe—on everyone who presents, whether they have symptoms or not. This "screening" is the result of attempts to diagnose disease before the symptoms appear. Theoretically this makes sense, but in fact the yield has been very low, partly because most diseases strike out of a clear blue sky, and secondly because screening normal people is boring and, because of the low yield, unrewarding; good doctors are too busy, and not interested enough in examining normal people, to take part. For this reason, interpretation of the findings, the most difficult part of screening, is not well done. This results in a great deal of anxiety and unnecessary referrals, which may outweigh the benefits. Screening of subgroups of the population for specific diseases, for example chest x-ray of food handlers, in contrast to screening the individual patient for many diseases, has a much higher yield, and the interpretation of the findings, because it is limited to one test, tends to be of a higher standard.

For the Record

Another factor which has encouraged the proliferation of unnecessary investigations is the fear that someone might conceivably ask for the results of them, and then the doctor who has failed to do them will appear to be incompetent. The daily electrocardiograms which chronicle the evolution of a cardiac infarction serve almost no function except that they are there if someone should ask. The ECG does not change until a moment or two before or after a complication sets in; if it needs monitoring, it needs constant monitoring, and the daily recording is not of much use. In some countries, not having done every conceivable investigation may be considered to be negligence by the courts.

Patterns of Practice

The amount of investigation required by an individual doctor depends on many factors. The less experienced need more confirmation. The more skilled the clinical examination and the better the judgement, the fewer the tests that are ordered. In some specialities the physical signs frequently allow a diagnosis to be made without recourse to tests, whereas others are much more dependent on tests. Our ability to test the function of the various systems is uneven. In the respiratory system, for example, almost every aspect of each component can be tested with precision and often non-invasively. In the central nervous system, the quantification of function is much less well developed.

The number of tests ordered by two doctors doing the same work will differ as a result of the interest they have in mechanisms, or in documenting changes for teaching purposes or for publication. Many excellent doctors are treatment orientated rather than mechanism orientated, and the tests which are used in the evaluation of treatment may not be the ones used for diagnosis.

Over-investigation

Over-investigation is, as Richard Asher says, a form of cruelty. Sometimes the habit of pursuing the diagnosis until it is established persists even when it is clear that the patient is too ill or too frail to have anything done about it. The criterion for ordering a test on a patient is whether you would have the test yourself if you were in his position. The desire to leave no stone unturned in a last-ditch attempt to make the patient better is understandable but it must be tempered by judicious cost-benefit analysis.

Sometimes the doctor is pressed to over-investigate by relatives who may not understand the cost to the patient. Relatives like to feel that "everything possible was done," but that satisfaction must not be obtained at the patient's expense.

"Test Use to Generate Income"

A paragraph in an otherwise excellent article on tests, in one of the best medical journals in the world, has this heading, and contains the following sentence: "The small office laboratories of the internist, paediatrician and family physician provide convenient sources of income to offset the high cost (and relatively low economic return) of talking to and examining patients." This is a spine-chilling statement. When ordering tests, financial gain is not a relevant consideration.

IS THE TEST WORTH WHILE?

When deciding whether or not to perform a particular test, many incommensurable values have to be added up in the doctor's mind, and as they are incommensurable, no truly rational answer can be arrived at. When ordering a test, you weigh up the cost to the patient in terms of the discomfort and danger of doing the test, against the dangers of not doing it. Another weight on the scales is the cost to other patients whose test or treatment may be delayed or impaired by performances of the test which you are considering. An investigation with a finite risk may reduce the risk of treatment, and investigative morbidity and mortality should be lumped together with the risk of medical or surgical treatment. An investigation with a finite mortality may reveal that a patient is unsuitable for an operation with a higher mortality, and here again that net gain must be considered in weighing the cost of investigation.

Although the weighing up process is complex, constant practice, the low risk rates, and the repeated reappearance of the same considerations, combine to make the process semi-automatic and rapid. When, however, a disaster occurs as the result of a test, the doctor dearly wishes that he had not ordered it whether it was necessary or not, but particularly of course if it was not. In ordering a test, therefore, the thought in the back of one's mind should be "If this test goes wrong, will my conscience be clear?," and secondly "If I had to give my reasons for ordering this test to a coroner, would I be absolutely certain of my ground?" The test should only be done if the answer to both questions is positive.

If, whenever you order or carry out a test, you try and forecast what the result will be on clinical grounds, you will sharpen your clinical acumen. Try and avoid the routine ordering of tests. Each time you order one, no matter how trivial, ask yourself why you are ordering it.

TELLING THE PATIENT ABOUT TESTS

You tell the patient enough about tests to satisfy his curiosity and allay his anxiety, taking great care that in so doing you do not inadvertently produce the opposite effect. If the tests are non-invasive or virtually risk free, they can be regarded simply as an extension of the physical examination, and all that you need or should say is that you are going to have them done, give an indication of what they are for and how unpleasant they will be, and tell the patient that you will talk with him about his condition when the test results are known.

When telling a patient about the test to which you are about to subject him, you should say what the tests are for—for example "to see if your kidney is working properly"—and then give an account of the amount of unpleasantness which is involved, rather than a technical explanation of what is being done. "No needles are involved" is always warmly appreciated. "This test involves three separate blood tests" or "It is about as unpleasant as going to the dentist" or "You will be given something to make you drowsy" are ways of describing the part of the test which is of most interest to the patient.

Investigation of Children

Children live in the present and they find it more difficult to take a long-term view than adults. The pain or unpleasantness which you are inflicting on them now, is not mitigated by the concept that it is all being done for their eventual good, and you must bear this in mind when telling them about tests.

How Much to Tell?

There are three aspects of tests which are of concern to the patient. The first is the nature of the test. Some of the tests which are now done routinely *sound* harrowing and dangerous. Indeed, when they were first proposed many of them were received with horror by the profession itself. We have gradually got used to them because we have learned that the risk is small. But the patient has not had this experience, and even if you explain to him that the test is not dangerous, he has to swallow, at a time when he is not at his best, what it has taken doctors years to get used to. This is an almost impossible feat, and it is the basis for my belief that the patient should be told as little as possible about the nature of the procedure if there is any chance that he will find the explanation frightening. He should be told enough to satisfy his curiosity, which if not satisfied, will breed anxiety. The test is after all being performed on him, and he has the "right" to know, but only if he wants to know, and only if he does not come to regret having asked. A large portion of the population would rather not know, and it is difficult for the healthy student or doctor to be certain quite what his own attitude would be if he were in the patient's position. The same rules of minimal disclosure of technicalities govern the investigation of sick doctors and nurses.

Discomfort

The patient's second concern is how much discomfort there will be. The normal range of both physical pain threshold and of stoicism entails that there are great differences in the degree of discomfort which patients will tolerate. Even venepuncture is unpleasant, and when you talk about investigations to friends who are healthy, they usually say that they could not bear to have *that* done to them. This is the reasonable attitude to unpleasantness, because the amount which you are prepared to suffer depends on how much you have to gain from the test, or how much you have to lose from not having it done. When you are fit, all tests are unacceptable unless they are non-invasive, and even these may be psychologically disturbing, for they may reveal an abnormality of which the subject is now bliss-fully unaware. The thought of a lumbar puncture or of liver biopsy is frightening to the fit and the unfit, but if you have a serious disease, the fear is mitigated by the desire to be cured, and if you know that the investigation is part of the cure, your attitude to it is quite differ-ent. It may be difficult for a healthy student or a doctor to under-stand this. Unless you have had a serious disease it is difficult to imagine how it disrupts life, and how fervently one wishes to be rid of it. "I could not bear to have that done to me" changes to "I would do anything to be free of this disease." Finally, one should be influ-enced by the fact, and tell the patient, that if the test is painful or frightening it is almost invariably done under local anaesthesia, or sedation or even general anaesthesia, and that these very largely nul-lify the unpleasantness. Unfortunately, sedation or anaesthesia may impair the quality of the findings.

Itemising the Discomforts

Minimal disclosure of technicalities is made more acceptable to the patient if he is given maximal forewarning of symptoms which he may feel during the test. A blow-by-blow description of what he may feel during the length of the procedure forewarns and forearms him. If he knows that a symptom may well develop, and if he is reassured that it will go away in so many minutes, he can bear it stoically. It is the duty of the doctor or auxiliary who does the test to say these things, as they are about to occur, but the doctor who orders the test should say them too, in case no one else does. It is unexpected discomfort which is difficult to tolerate. If you tell the patient that he will feel a tickling sensation in his abdomen, it may persuade him that what he feels is not discomfort. Whoever does the test should announce in advance any event, no matter how trivial, that the patient will notice. If reassurance is given from the beginning, and in advance, the patient gradually realises that he is not going to be taken by surprise.

Risks

The patient's third and least concern is risk. People do not associate tests with risk in the way that they associate surgery with risk. This attitude to risk is both fortunate and fitting, because the patient gains nothing by worry about the risk and the proper doctor has shoulders broad enough to bear the worry for the patient. The doctor who orders a test must have the risk in the forefront of his mind, to a degree which is actually disproportionate to the risk involved. Most tests carry low risk, otherwise they would not be done, but when you order or perform a test you must wonder whether this patient is going to be the one in a thousand, or in ten thousand, who dies as a result of it.

I do not tell patients about the risks of investigations, except on the rare occasions when they ask, and then I give not a figure from the statistics, but an everyday analogy such as "There is about the same chance of something going wrong during this test as there is of your being knocked down by a bus on your way home from the hospital." Neither a statistic nor an analogy is relevant to the individual patient who either suffers the complication or avoids it, but such an analogy, delivered with conviction, looking the patient in the eye and letting him understand that you are willing to go into more detail if he requires it, is usually enough to settle the question of risk in his mind. If he is unsatisfied, you may say that the risk to him of not having the investigation is much greater than the risk of the test. Or you may tell him that about ten of these tests are carried out in your hospital every day, "and we have never had any problem." People derive much comfort from thinking that they are one of many. What they do not want to know is that one in ten thousand dies from the anaesthetic or that, in his case, his poor physical condition makes the risk quite substantial. This subject is discussed in more detail in Chapter 7.

Telling the patient as *little* as possible about risk does not mean as *briefly* as possible, and a leisurely, limited explanation is more satisfying than a brief, revealing one. Judgement is needed to see how much more the patient would like to hear before he feels satisfied.

A Resolute Attitude to the Patient's Risk

They say that when a surgeon declares "I'll risk it," he means that the patient will risk it. Although the patient does in fact take the risk, a proper doctor feels as if he is taking the risk himself, and does unto others only that which he would advise for himself. Once you have decided that a test is necessary, then it has to be done, regardless of its risks and discomforts, because the decision is based on the premise that it would be more dangerous not to do it. Your attitude when you describe the test to the patient is based on its inevitability and on the need to assure the patient that it is not more than acceptably unpleasant. On no account must any lingering doubt that you have about your decision, or about the extra risk in his case, be transmitted to the patient. Nor must your understandable reluctance to cause discomfort deflect you from your course. The doctor who "takes a chance" and fails to bronchoscope a colleague who has had a haemoptysis has been misled by his kindliness.

"I Saw It on Television"

The sick pay a high price for the enthusiasm with which television exploits the voyeurism of the general public. Sometimes a patient who has seen a television programme on the subject or who has a friend with a similar condition will ask "Does this mean that I will have a piece of my liver sucked out doctor?"—which must be a source of anxiety to anyone who has to have it done. You have to make sure that the patient realises that the test which you propose is a routine procedure, that the dangers of doing it are less than the risk to him of you not having the information, and that the discomfort involved is "about as bad as going to the dentist." On no account must you deny what is in fact going to be done, although you may wish to phrase it differently.

THE ACTUAL INVESTIGATION

A description of investigations is outside the scope of this book, but there are two general points which are important. The first is that although the person who performs the test is familiar with what goes on, the patient is not, and copious explanation of practical details of what you are about to do should be provided. You tell him that you are going to put some cold stuff on his arm, and then you say that you are injecting, through a small needle, some local anaesthetic which may sting. You say that he is to stand on this platform which can be made to move, and then you say that you will warn him before it starts to move, and so on. You can never assume that the patient will know what is going to happen. André Cournand, who won the Nobel prize for his work in cardiac and respiratory physiology, once visited our laboratory and asked if he could try the treadmill. We assumed that he would need no instruction. When the machine was started he was thrown off the platform, and was bruised and extremely annoyed.

The second general point about tests is that you should know exactly what you are going to do and do it skilfully. Patients measure the excellence of students and young doctors by the skill with which they perform tests. No technique is so trivial that you can afford to do it badly. Aim to enter all veins at the first attempt; if it is necessary to make two attempts you should feel a sense of professional failure, no matter how "difficult" the veins are. And similarly with all other techniques and tests. You must familiarise yourself with all the details of the test and the apparatus before the patient is brought in. The doctor who has the instruction manual in one hand and a scalpel in the other saps the patient's confidence. Discussion about which wire is which, or where the switch is, should be confined to times when the patient is not present. Patients often remember hearing discussions which took place when they were lightly anaesthetised.

"Are You All Right?"

After an intervention which may have untoward effects, it is natural and social good manners to ask the patient if he is all right. The more dangerous the intervention, the more likely is the tone of voice you use in this question to betray your anxiety. If everyone who enters the laboratory asks the same question, the patient begins to expect not to feel all right. If the untoward effect which you are expecting can be monitored, your question should be answered, before it is asked, by a glance at the screen. If it is not monitored, a look at the patient will tell you if he is all right or not. Assume that the patient is all right until you have evidence to the contrary. It is better to say "That's good" than "Are you all right?" Often the worst part of the procedure, from the patient's point of view, occurs early in the investigation. It is positively therapeutic to say to the patient "You'll be glad to hear that the worst part of the test is over." Quite often the relief of tension is almost palpable.

WHEN THINGS GO WRONG

Tests can be vitiated by events like power cuts, which are outside the control of the investigator, or they may be useless because someone has failed to do his job properly. In both circumstances the patient will have been put through "all that discomfort for nothing," and a proper professional ensures that all steps are taken before and during the investigation to reduce the chance of failure to a minimum. Whatever the cause of the failure, the doctor has to make up his mind whether the test should be repeated or not. If the test was unpleasant or dangerous, and if it has been spoiled for some reason, there is a tendency to feel that the patient has already "paid" for that test, and that it should not be done again. But as the reason for ordering the test in the first place was that the patient would be safer with it than without it, the logic of the situation demands that it be done again, except in those rare circumstances when the patient is thought to be too frail to survive a repetition of the test.

Making Your Excuses

Great care must be taken when explaining to a patient that a test has to be repeated. Any explanation will result in some loss of confidence. If the failure was due to a power cut, it raises the possibility that there may be another power cut on the second occasion. If you say that you will have your own generator ready he may wonder why it was not ready last time. If the explanation for the failure is that some member of the team forgot to load the camera, he will wonder what sort of a team he has got involved with, and what sort of mistake will be made next time. It is of the utmost importance for the future treatment of the patient that he should feel he is on a smooth production line where mistakes do not happen, so that he can place himself in the hands of the team, in the confidence that although mistakes happen, they happen elsewhere. This unrealistic level of confidence is an enormous aid to proper treatment, and the air of efficiency in the best hospitals sustains the patients.

In the circumstances, it seems justifiable to disguise the need for repetition wherever possible by pretending that a different test is to be done. It is not true, but no useful purpose is served by creating doubt in the patient's mind. When it is not possible to disguise the fact that the test is being repeated, the explanation which is least damaging to the patient's confidence should be given, regardless of what the true reason is. These false explanations are in no way given to lessen the investigator's legal or moral responsibilities. On the contrary, the investigator should regard any avoidable failure as a failure in professionalism which is unforgiveable.

When Things Go Wrong with the Patient

If some previously undescribed complication occurs as a result of a test, the doctor who ordered it must take that into account when he orders the test on another patient.

If a recognised complication occurs, the fact that it has happened to one of your patients should not bias you against the test. A theoretical mortality of one in a thousand is less shocking than the actual death of one patient in the thousand who you have investigated, or on whom you have ordered the investigation. It is difficult to avoid being uneasy next time you perform the same investigation, but it is essential to try and keep the true mortality and morbidity in perspective, rather than to be stampeded into abandoning a useful procedure whose risk had been taken into account before it was ordered.

THE PATIENT WHO REFUSES TO HAVE A TEST DONE

It is every patient's right to refuse to have a test, and it is every doctor's duty to explain to the patient that the refusal has a certain risk, to be quite certain that the patient understands this risk, and to try and persuade him to change his mind. This must be done in a doctorly, unthreatening, understanding way. The patient may have very good reasons for refusing, and it is best to ask him what these are at the outset and try and counter them. If the patient has a friend or relative who died during a test which the patient thinks is similar to the one which you are advising, he will need to be convinced that the risk of the test in his case is less than the risk of treatment without it. If refusal of the test makes it impossible for you to continue with treatment, the patient must be made to understand this. Often the test is desirable but not essential, and the doctor must be as accommodating as he possibly can, without putting himself in an indefensible position.

THE INTERPRETATION OF TESTS

Few tests are infallible. There is almost always the possibility of mechanical or human error even when things are automated, and this possibility is greater when human interpretation is required. Many tests can be done badly or well, and sometimes the test results are vitiated by some factor in the patient (excitement or pain for example) or by some factor in the procedure (for example inexpert anaesthesia may alter the function which is being investigated). All these things have to be borne in mind when the test is being interpreted. Sometimes tests are unsatisfactory when the disease is severe. A badly damaged kidney may not concentrate urine well enough to give a pyelogram which can be reliably interpreted. Patients have great faith in tests and it is difficult to persuade them that the test has not provided an unequivocal answer.

Doctors who order tests often have to rely on someone else for the interpretation, but in some situations they may be able to interpret the test themselves. For example, an experienced orthopaedic surgeon's interpretation of a bone x-ray may well be better than that of a general radiologist. A report is only as good as the man who makes it. In other situations the doctor who orders the test can have no valid opinion about the interpretation. If, however, the result of the test does not fit with the clinical diagnosis, much is to be gained by talking to the person who performed the test, in order to find out how much reliance should be placed on the findings. The typewritten test results may carry more conviction than the investigator feels. All tests have snags which the person who does them knows about. His confidence in his result will vary from one test to another, and if you discuss the test with him you will be able to gauge whether he is confident, or overconfident, in his findings. People who do tests do not like to be challenged about them, particularly if the questioner is ill-informed, but they are usually willing to discuss the snags if they are approached in the right way. The healthy scepticism which one feels about tests, particularly the tests done at St. Elsewhere's, should not be apparent to the tester or the tested.

The Normal Range

One has to have a flexible attitude to the concept of the normal range. Firstly, the tails of the bell extend to infinity at either end.

Secondly, a value which is within the normal range may be abnormal for the patient concerned. I once looked after a patient who had several relapses of pulmonary tuberculosis. When he was well, his erythrocyte sedimentation rate was always 2 or 3 mm in the first hour. When he relapsed, it rose to 7 or 8 mm, well within the normal range. Finally, the range of normals may have been determined on an inadequate or quite inappropriate sample of "normals." "Normal" values often vary greatly between one laboratory and another.

TELLING THE PATIENT ABOUT THE RESULTS OF THE TESTS

Favourable Results

Test results should be relayed to the patient as quickly as possible. If the result of the test is favourable, that is to say if the result is the one which both patient and doctor hoped for, there is little problem in communicating the result. The only caveat is that only those results which are known with certainty should be reported. For example, a surgeon who takes a biopsy from a mass which he believes to be malignant may, once he has removed it, be "certain" from its appearance that it is benign. It is better, however, to wait for the histological findings before the patient is reassured. Often a test result stimulates a patient to ask if this means such-and-such. The answer should not go beyond the facts which have been established. If the doctor feels that there is nothing wrong with the patient, and has had the test done to exclude any lingering doubts that he or the patient may have had, then normal findings must be treated as if this meant that no disease is present, and the patient should be told about it unequivocally and joyfully.

The knowledge that a test may not be sensitive enough to detect mild or early disease makes some doctors adopt a mealy-mouthed attitude to normal findings; "Well, there is nothing there at the moment," or "We haven't been able to show anything abnormal," reinforces old doubts and sows the seeds of new ones. Such words are translations of N.A.D.; the patient wants to hear that nothing abnormal is present. Nothing abnormal *demonstrated* may simply mean that it has escaped detection. If you say "I'm glad to say that your chest x-ray is normal" or "your result is like that of someone half your age" you take therapeutic advantage of the patient's faith in tests. (The question of reassurance is gone into in depth in Chapter 7.) Clearly, if the test is normal but there is strong clinical suspicion that it has failed to detect disease, further tests must be done and reassurance must be withheld until more evidence has been obtained. Even in these circumstances it is helpful to remark, wherever possible, that as the test is normal, any abnormality, if present, cannot be very severe or important.

It is when the doctor is not sure whether he is right in his view that the patient is normal that he is most likely to sit on the fence when he is faced with normal findings. Uncertainty or inexperience are loads which the doctor must carry, and he must resist the temptation to insure against error by hedging his bets.

Unfavourable Results

If the test results are unfavourable, there is often no need to communicate them to the patient. If several tests have been done and only one has a result which is unfavourable, there is no point in telling the patient about it unless his ignorance of the result would interfere with his treatment. Sometimes a bad result can be looked at from the bright side with a better therapeutic result. If the test shows that the disease has progressed too far for any operative treatment, for example, then the statement "I'm afraid that this is inoperable" is not nearly as therapeutic as "You will be better off without surgery" or even "You will be glad to hear that you do not have to have the operation." Human ability for self-deception is unlimited and it can be turned into a potent therapeutic tool.

FILING OF RESULTS

Reports of tests, and indeed the recordings obtained during the test, frequently get lost. The records must be carefully stored whenever possible and the reports must be incorporated in the patient's notes, making quite certain from the patient's name, sex, age and number that the test results are appropriately filed. When reading test results from the notes it is worth training yourself to glance automatically at the identification section before you read the result. When looking at x-rays or reports of tests, the possibility that they refer to a different patient should always be in the back of one's mind. X-rays are sometimes numbered with the patient's date of birth, and although the odds are very much against it, I have had two patients with the same first name, surname and date of birth. Fortunately, the shape of the chest of the patient I had just examined was unusual, and the x-ray with his name and date of birth on it could not have "belonged" to him. If a test or a result shows a sudden and unexpected change, or does not fit with the clinical findings, the possibility that it refers to another patient should be examined.

6. ON THE ART OF DIAGNOSIS

THE LOGICAL BASIS OF DIAGNOSIS

The nature of the logical processes involved in diagnosis is itself intrinsically interesting, and it would be of great benefit to students if the processes could be analysed and described. A number of clinicians who are interested in logic and philosophy have attempted to describe the processes, but like the electrical analogues used to explain haemodynamic phenomena, the language of philosophy is difficult to understand. In fact, it seems easier for those who are not used to handling philosophical concepts to grasp the nature of diagnosis than to understand the language of philosophy which is required to describe it.

PATTERN RECOGNITION

Until the turn of the century, diagnosis was made by the process of pattern recognition. Just as a botanist identifies a flower by matching its characteristics to a textbook description, so the doctor would assess the symptoms and signs and compare them with the textbook description of the disease. Diseases rarely fit their descriptions exactly, and the symptoms and signs frequently resemble those of other diseases, so the probabilities were narrowed down to the differential diagnosis. The skill lay in choosing the right one. And herein lies the danger of the method, for the same pattern can often be produced by several diseases, or by diseases in combination.

Teachers used to combat the bad habit of making several diagnoses in the same patient to explain away all the symptoms and signs, by frequent advocacy of Ockham's Razor. This is a philosophical concept which advocates trying to find a single cause whenever possible. The usual overswing of the pendulum resulted in one disease being diagnosed when two were present. After all, it is only twice as unlikely that a patient will have two diseases as it is that he will have one. As an example, wheezing in a patient with heart disease may be due to cardiac failure or it may be due to asthma. It may be due to asthma even if he has not had asthma before.

Diagnosis by pattern recognition was, and is, extremely valuable, firstly because we are all so good at it. A glimpse of the back of the head of a colleague as he turns into a doorway at the end of a long corridor is enough to identify him. Secondly, we still lack a clear understanding of mechanism in some of the diseases of most systems. In some systems, notably the skin and the mind, knowledge of mechanisms is so imperfect that the pattern recognition approach is the rule.

When biochemical, histological and haematological tests became available, these too were used for pattern recognition, and their usefulness did not depend on understanding. In tuberculosis, for example, no one knew why the erythrocyte sedimentation rate was raised, but nevertheless it was an extremely useful piece of evidence in that diagnosis. We have a vast amount of information on the range of findings in most diseases. When the norms have been properly established and the routine measurements are meticulously performed, the knowledge that 80 per cent of all patients with so-and-so's disease give a positive reaction to a certain test, or have a value over such-and-such, is extremely useful and is hard data.

THE PHYSIOLOGICAL APPROACH

In this century there has been enormous development of our under-standing of the causes and mechanism of many diseases. The tools which were used to investigate physiology are now used to evaluate the pathophysiology of disease in the individual patient, and the modern doctor is trained to think in terms of disordered function or disordered anatomy. Thus, if a patient has diplopia, whereas for-merly one would have summoned up a list of causes of that condi-tion, one nowadays prefers to think of the function of binocular vision and to picture a lesion, of no matter what nature, which could upset that system. When you have done that with all the symptoms and signs, the diagnosis is made on the basis of finding a disease pro-cess which is known to cause that particular combination of defects. You still have to have a list of causes, so there is no escape from parrot-fashion learning.

When we come to understand all disease processes, the pattern recognition approach will die out, but at present our understanding of mechanisms is not nearly as complete as the teaching in the phys-iology department would lead one to believe. Indeed, the modern student tends to be so mechanism-minded that he rejects any unex-plained phenomenon regardless of its diagnostic or therapeutic po-tential. When you tell him, for example, that syphilis of the nervous system causes general paralysis of the insane in mesomorphs and tabes in ectomorphs, his face lights up with interest. When, in reply to his question, you tell him that no one knows why this is so, you can see from his eyes that he has filed that one away under "anec-dotes," a category with pejorative overtones, and the purveyor of such "old wives' tales" loses face. Think about mechanisms whenever they are relevant, but do not disdain pattern recognition when they are not.

GOODNESS OF FIT: THE BASIS OF PATTERN RECOGNITION

You suspect at first glance that a patient has rheumatic fever because in some way he reminds you of a patient you saw some time ago who had it. If asked to describe the face of rheumatic fever, you would be unable to do so, but if the patient does have rheumatic fever your diagnosis cannot be described as a guess. It is not intuition either. It is pattern recognition of so subtle a kind that you cannot describe it. This inexplicable and accurate assessment of the goodness of fit of sensory input is present at all levels of complexity. When we recognise notable goodness of fit we experience a surge of pleasure, which confirms the diagnosis of goodness of fit. All our senses can produce this effect. Visual, auditory, gustatory or intellectual harmony excites one person more than another, possibly on the basis of the discriminatory capacity of the organ concerned. If you are colour blind you are unlikely to find any pleasure in seeing someone wearing shoes, stockings and a skirt of different but harmonious colours. If on the other hand you are sensitive to small differences of colour, such a sight is unexpectedly and disproportionately pleasurable. The usual bell-shaped distribution of the quality of each of the sense organs ensures that each of us has a mixed bag of these faculties. You may, for example, be exceptionally good at matching colours but tone deaf. Doctors need to be more than two standard deviations above the mean for intellectual discrimination of goodness of fit.

We recognise people and places and the bark of our own dog, but we cannot teach these skills to anyone else by description alone. We assemble ingredients and cook dishes which, by general agreement, taste delicious. Mozart assembled notes in a way which is pleasing to those who like music and have been brought up in the Western tradition. The music can be recognised as his even if it has not been heard before. Art historians detect fakes because the goodness of fit is not quite perfect. Most of the important decisions in life are taken on similar grounds. You take up medicine, or fall in love, or decide to practise surgery for reasons which are neither measurable nor easily defined. The reasons which you offer when asked may not be the actual reasons for your choice, even if you think they are. Advice to a patient, which may involve one of the most important decisions in his life, is arrived at in the same way and is as difficult to justify and explain.

Yet despite the nature of our data base, two sensible doctors, trained in the traditions of Western medicine, will usually come to the same decision about what to do about a particular patient. Sometimes one will favour one treatment more than the other, but they will not regard each other's solutions as ridiculous. Doctors often disagree, and sometimes this is because one or the other is not properly trained or has poor judgement. Sometimes there is disagreement because there is no clear understanding of how the disease ought to be treated and no one knows whether this or that treatment is better than doing nothing at all. But in the vast area where effective treatment is available, there is little room for disagreement except on matters of detail.

Cerebral Bioassay

Our system of coming to conclusions works well, and the fact that it can be explained only in part is the reason why medicine is more an art than a science. In those situations where our motivation is unclear to ourselves, we cannot explain it to others, nor can we make a quantitative estimate of the reasons for our conclusions. For this reason doctors have been browbeaten into feeling that because the decision-making process cannot be measured—and for this reason is not scientific—it must be worse. This is a fallacy. A piece of muscle in an organ bath will respond to drugs at levels undetectable by any chemical or physical assay, with the result that bioassay is often a hundred times as sensitive as chemical assay. Similarly the goodness of fit capability of the human mind—cerebral bioassay—is incomparably better than any scientific test. We do not understand exactly how the muscle contracts, but that does not make the bioassay any less accurate.

THE IMPORTANCE OF "MECHANISMS"

The knowledge that a certain lesion usually produces that symptom or sign is extremely useful even if we do not understand how the function was controlled in health, or how it was modified by disease. Until recently physicians were happy to leave it at that, because there was so little effective treatment. With the advent of new and powerful drugs, however, the call for "rational" treatment has produced a profession which wants to know how both the system and the drug works. We like to explain why drug A works better than drug B, and we no longer feel that all that is required is to find out by trial which drug is superior.

If we understood how an effect was produced, and how disease impaired its efficiency, we could design drugs to counteract the disease. It has to be stressed, however, that this is our eventual aim and not our current achievement. In the 1980s we still do not understand how digitalis works. Indeed, although Withering wrote a book about it in 1785, and literally millions of doses of it must have been administered since, there is today hot controversy over whether it has any sustained inotropic effect on the diseased heart.

ATTITUDE TO INFORMATION

The profession is inundated with information both in the journals and from the pharmaceutical industry. Much of this information is contradictory or seems not to make sense, and the individual doctor has to have opinions on matters which are extremely difficult to judge. In addition to the written word, opinions for or against some hypothesis or treatment pass from mouth to mouth. In a book like this it is not possible to do more than suggest an overall approach to new information. The profession is usually pictured as being unwilling to accept anything new. This may well have been true in the past, but at present the pendulum has swung to the other extreme, and the profession in general is too gullible. Cynicism is cheap and easy and inadvisable, but a healthy scepticism, based firmly on the short half-life of medical views, should condition your approach to the nostra which are purveyed. Above all, new ideas should be subjected to the searchlight of common-sense before they are accepted, and even then it is necessary to bear in mind that for every view which is expressed someone has "evidence" which supports the opposite view. Extremism in medicine has a very poor track record. *Festina lente*.

INCOMMENSURABLE VALUES

It is difficult to weigh things against one another even when they can be weighed accurately. It is impossible to say whether a pound of salt is "better" than a pound of sugar, even if the price is the same. It depends which you need. In more complicated issues, comparison is even more difficult. For example, we can grade symptoms, but moderate (grade 2) dyspnoea cannot be compared with grade 2 angina. We can say that an aortic valve is stenosed or regurgitant and that the degree of malfunction in each case is moderate. If the valve is both stenosed and regurgitant we may say that the dominant lesion is regurgitation. But aortic stenosis is one disease, with one set of sequelae, and aortic regurgitation has different sequelae. So when we say that the patient has dominant regurgitation we are saying that in the natural course of this patient's disease, although the valve is stenosed, the evolution will be mainly that of regurgitation. But whether the left ventricular dilatation and back pressure effects of regurgitation are "worse" or "better" than the angina and sudden death of stenosis, is another question.

MAKING THE DIAGNOSIS

When a client complained to Whistler that he had charged a high price for a portrait which had been completed in half an hour, the painter replied that the portrait was the product of a lifetime's experience. Diagnosis is like that too. You bring to bear on it your self and your knowledge and your attitudes. Diagnosis thus starts long before you see a patient. While taking the history, doing the examination and ordering investigations, the process of diagnosis is proceeding steadily and if you are skilled, careful and honest, the diagnosis, if you are ever going to make it, will be making itself. In accounting, you list all the figures and add them up at the end. In diagnosis you are adding from the beginning, and aiming at producing a portrait of disease, and when your task is to exclude disease, your portrait reveals the imposture. Whilst you diagnose optimistically, always hoping for the least bad, your honesty will ensure that you do not flinch from diagnosing a disease you wish the patient did not have.

7. ADVICE AND EXPLANATION

DECIDING WHAT ADVICE TO GIVE

THE PATIENT consults you because he wants your advice about his symptoms, and if you adopt the therapeutic approach to history-taking and physical examination, you keep the therapeutic implication of each symptom and sign in the front of your mind. This certainly does not mean that you treat each symptom and sign with a specific remedy. Quite the contrary, the treatment of symptoms without a search for their cause can be extremely dangerous, as epitomised by the patient whose anaemia is treated with iron until it becomes evident that its cause is a carcinoma of the colon. All the findings mould your view of the severity of the disease and hence determine how far you are prepared to go in treatment.

Responsibility for the advice which he gives lies squarely on the shoulders of the clinician, and each decision should be able to withstand the scrutiny of his peers. There is almost always more than one way in which the patient can be treated, and even when only one line of therapy is available, there is always the alternative of doing nothing. The nature and extent of the disease and its risks and complications are one weight in the cerebral scales. This weight is modified by the physical and mental condition of the patient. On the other pan of the scales come the risks and complications of the treatment under consideration.

The Highest Common Factor

The trained and experienced doctor puts himself, or his nearest and dearest, in the patient's position, and asks himself what he would do if he were advising himself or his family. He gives the same advice to the patient. No other advice is acceptable; no other is justifiable. Patients are delighted to hear that this is the basis of your advice. As in the case of investigations, the criterion for going ahead is whether your conscience is clear, and whether you feel that you would have no difficulty in defending your action to your peers. William Evans said that no patient should be the worse for seeing a doctor, and this minimum requirement is far from being met.

The Weighing Up

When a doctor weighs the pros and cons of what advice to give to Mrs. Jones, although he takes into account all that he can discover about her and her disease, he is not literally weighing things up and acting on the final figure. Often the decision is not difficult at all. If she has anaemia due to malabsorption of iron, for which no cause has been found, the doctor knows that untreated she will deteriorate or even die and that if iron is prescribed she will get better. There is of course a risk in taking iron tablets. There is a risk in taking anything, if it is only the risk of having to regard oneself as a patient, a person who is not healthy. But the dangers of taking iron are infinitesimal compared with the risks and disadvantages of doing nothing, and any sane person would agree on what to do. The risks of treatment vary from barely worth considering to considerable, and this risk must be weighed against the risk of doing nothing. The more sensitive the balance, the more it is affected by tiny differences between the two pans. If the balance is crude, a kilogram or two of difference is necessary to make the scales come down on one side or the other; if it is sensitive, a milligram will be enough.

The doctor's cerebral weighing machine may be good, bad or indifferent. Its sensitivity depends on common-sense, which probably cannot be learned, information about the patient, which depends on technique and diligence, and on knowledge of disease, which may be improved by study.

The Nature of Your Conclusion

The doctor has to make up his mind about the diagnosis and the treatment by "weighing up" many factors which are not actually weighable. His conclusion is not one an engineer would make, but rather a collage of fragments which he arranges to make a picture which seems to him to suit the situation best. Many doctors are not aware of the unscientific nature of their decisions.

Very often the decision is so obvious that it is hardly necessary to consider it as weighing up; it is going on throughout the history-taking and the examination. In these circumstances, little or no judgement is required. At other times the contents of the pans have to be scrutinised.

The Patient's View

The general public does not realise that medicine is an "art," like cooking. Decades of "breakthroughs," "wonder drugs" and television programmes showing white-coated miracle workers in their space fiction laboratories have produced a distorted picture. This, and the certainty with which doctors express their opinions in the media, have given the population the feeling that the subject is like physics, and that only a few problems remain to be solved. After all, if you can manipulate an unmanned space craft on the moon from earth, surely you can tell whether or not a man has a lesion in his midbrain.

The emphasis on positive health and routine check-ups, has served to foster the illusion that provided you catch it early, you can put it right. Early diagnosis sometimes facilitates a cure, but for is-chaemic heart disease or neoplasms or neurological diseases or the common cold, namely most of the diseases which are important, it does not make a great deal of difference.

An Attitude to Death

This is not a book about medical ethics, which is a thorny, intensely personal and ever-changing subject. However, the question of a doctor's attitude to death is germane to advice-giving, and without going into questions of belief or strongly held feelings about whether or not it is "right" to take this or that action, I would like to put what I think of as the contra-statistical attitude.

"Threescore years and ten" are now the average expectation of life, and each year this figure is pushed slightly higher, not because the old are living very much longer, but because the young are not dying in such large numbers, and thus a higher proportion of people reach old age. Nevertheless, "In the midst of life we are in death."

Most people die suddenly as a result of accident or disease, and sudden death is no respecter of prognosis. Neither is exceptional longevity. In the individual patient, the odds are irrelevant. A certain therapy may be effective in one patient in four, or in a hundred or even in a thousand; but if it cures the patient, both of you will be pleased with its efficacy. Conversely, it is of little satisfaction to the patient or his doctor to know that the particular complication which has developed is rare. For the patient it was 100 per cent. Whilst one bases one's operational philosophy on probabilities and analysis of the outcome in other patients, one has constantly to bear in mind that outcome too has a bell-shaped distribution, that the standard deviation may be larger than the mean, and that the patient under consideration may be outside three standard deviations from the mean, in either direction. This means that the individual patient may die very quickly or he may have a normal expectation of life.

Assessment of Risks and Complications

When the risk is appreciable, we weigh it up, but our emotions and personal—not necessarily representative—experience play a large part in our decision. If the last two patients who had that treatment did badly, it affects your judgement, even though the next twenty may do well. You have to guard against over-reacting to recent experience. Although your advice is largely the result of a combination of what is reported to be the case and your own experience, the risks vary in the individual case. Few doctors have enough experience of the diseases which they treat to be able to assess accurately the risk in a particular patient. If the mortality from some large series is 2 per cent for the therapy which you recommend, this does not mean that the risk for this particular patient who is old and has mild diabetes as well as the condition which you propose to treat is 2 per cent. The 2 per cent figure may have been arrived at by including every sort of lesion in patients of all ages and throughout the range of physical fitness, or alternatively, all the patients in the series may have been young and in good general health. For the patient in front of you, the percentage mortality or morbidity cannot be accurately assessed. Even if it could be accurately assessed it would be difficult to put it on the cerebral scales, because mortality and morbidity in the individual patient is an all-or-none phenomenon: the patient either gets the complication, or he doesn't. It is difficult to ascribe weights to the possibilities that he *will* be better but he *may* be dead, particularly when the disease for which he is being treated does not threaten his life. In estimating the risk, it is easy to forget that for both medical and surgical treatment the skill of the author of the series may not be the same as your own.

A further difficulty in weighing up is that the patient himself would not be able to say in any authoritative way whether he would rather have the disease or the complication of treatment. Although he has experience of the disease, which the doctor is unlikely to have, he has no experience of the complication. For example, the pain of claudication can be excruciating. Operation may, if it goes wrong, result in loss of the limb. Who can say whether it is preferable to keep your own painful leg or to have an artificial limb, which after training may enable you to walk for miles in relative comfort? To some patients, the loss of a limb would be so horrifying that they would rather not take the risk, and would find life perfectly acceptable if they were pain free when walking about the house, if necessarily slowly. If the patient had led a sedentary life, if he lived in a flat with a lift, and possessed suitable transport, his way of life need hardly be limited. If, however, the patient's pleasure came from walking or sightseeing, an artificial limb becomes a much more acceptable proposition. Whilst it is true that the operation is usually successful, in recommending it the doctor must give excessive weight to the complications.

A Plan of Campaign

Having made up your mind which treatment would suit the patient best, you then think about the details of the programme by which you will achieve this end. The exact course of treatment will be influenced by new findings and the patient's response to therapy, but the clearer your mental picture of your broad strategy, the more effective will be your advice.

Changing Your Advice

A proper doctor is ready to change course if at any time this seems to be necessary. You may want to change the treatment because it has been ineffective or only partially effective or if it has untoward side effects. Patients are willing to accept that you did what you thought best in the first instance, and that events have shown that the treatment was not satisfactory. They understand that now you are going to prescribe what you think best in the light of your observation of his response.

Learning from Experience

If the patient is harmed by taking your advice, you may feel that what has occurred is one of the known complications which you took into account when recommending the treatment, and that if presented with the same problem again, your advice would be exactly the same. If, however, the complication is unexpected, it will have to be put in the balance when next you consider a similar problem. Learning from experience is made more difficult because patients and their diseases are so varied that the outcome in an individual patient is uncertain. Frequently, the patient will or will not get better regardless of what you do. In those cases where the doctor's judgement plays an important role in the outcome, it is difficult for even the most sensible doctor to know whether the outcome in a particular patient would have been different if he had acted differently. It is particularly difficult to know this when you do not have much judgement.

There is no external assessor. The opinion of patients is misleading because they confuse kindness, the amount of time the doctor spends with them and a successful outcome, with excellence. For all these reasons the feedback, which is so important for learning, is usually not available. Furthermore, if nobody is in a position to monitor your performance, it is easy to imagine that you are actually doing rather well.

Ill-advised Advice

Doctors are often asked, or may volunteer, their advice on subjects on which they are not qualified to give opinions. The fact that many years ago you spent three months "doing" midwifery does not mean that your opinion about the Leboyer method is any better than that of an equally intelligent layman, particularly if the layman has personal experience of the method. "Doctors for nuclear disarmament" should carry about the same weight as "Musicians for nuclear disarmament." Limit your advice to those subjects in which you have expertise, or if you are forced to give an opinion, make it clear that you speak without special knowledge. If doctors give bad advice, it impairs the acceptance of their good advice.

THE CONSULTATION

Role-Playing in Advice-Giving

In advice-giving, role-playing reaches its apogee. Truths, half truths and statistics have to be welded together into an instrument to make the patient better. Like a magician's trick, if you can see how it is done, it is not magic; undetectable role-playing is a boon to the patient and the hallmark of the complete clinician. Your stance must tell the patient that you understand—and will manage—the physical, psychological and socio-economic aspects of his disease.

At the beginning of this book, I said that one of the main reasons for dressing like a doctor, behaving like a doctor and acting the role during the consultation, was to establish in the patient's mind that you were worthy of the considerable trust which he has to have in you in order to take your advice. What is advised may be painful or frightening, or it may involve giving up some favourite occupation like smoking or drinking or exercise or eating or work. The doctor who advises a Head of State that he must resign on medical grounds must be very convincing if his advice is to be taken.

Giving Advice Wholeheartedly

Once you have come down on one side or the other in a difficult decision, and perhaps taken advice, or waited a while for things to settle in your mind, then you must take the course which is indicated with total commitment. You know that the scales are inaccurate, that your decision has large unconfirmable components, and that a small change in any one of the components might have brought you to a different conclusion. It may be only a microgram of difference which has made you take course A rather than course B, but a sensitive balance comes down firmly on the heavier side, and stays there. The proper doctor acts as if there were no other course than the one he has advised, or rather as if the one which he advises is clearly the best course. The patient badly needs this feeling that the advice is wholehearted, whether it be a question of treatment or of reassurance that he is normal. William Evans, who first described the placebo effect, said that to get full benefit from it, advice must be given enthusiastically.

The way decisions are arrived at make it necessary to play a role when giving advice. Your doubts must not be allowed to show through. The doctor who tells the patient that he cannot make up his mind whether to do operation A or operation B is no doctor. Naturally, different methods of treatment suit different patients, but this must be taken into account during the weighing up process. The patient cannot imagine the two operations and perform comparative cost-benefit analysis. This is true even when the patient is a doctor in another speciality. Most doctors who are ill put themselves in the hands of someone they trust, and then they do exactly as they are told. Most patients have to make sure that they do trust you, and then they want to be treated in the same way.

The Over-balanced View

I was once a registrar on a Medical Unit at a time when all the senior members of the team were more scientific than doctorly. Fair minded, intelligent, listening to all sorts of opinions and treating them seriously, they would present rather tentative views to the patient. Each time we visited the bedside of a nice old lady who had a hiatus hernia which was ulcerated, we dithered. We presented first one side and then the other to her and weighed, over and over, the risks and advantages of medical treatment compared with the risks and advantages of surgery. The pendulum swung from one view to the other and back and the patient looked sadder and sadder. Finally, we asked for a surgical opinion. The surgeon arrived, with a huge retinue in formation behind him. Tall, elegant, steely-eyed and with a speckling of grey in his immaculately barbered hair, he marched straight up to her and said "Madam, your stomach's in your chest and furthermore it's ulcerated. I shall put it all right, half past two on Thursday." "Oh thank you doctor" she cried and her face lit up. Here at last was a doctor who knew what to do. She never looked back, and I learned the importance of appearing confident whether or not that confidence is justified.

An Attitude to Life

We are not very good at forecasting outcome. Firstly there is the range of severity within a particular disease. Then there is the variation in human response to disease, both physical and psychological. The will to fight the disease can lead to "miracles" of survival. Finally there are the errors of diagnosis, coupled with the pathetic inadequacy of our knowledge. The world is full of eighty-year-old aunties who were told that they had "weak chests" and that they would not live a normal lifespan. Modern equivalents of weak chests abound. The diagnoses are more precise, but the accuracy of prognosis is about the same. In the individual patient who confronts you, in the face of all these likelihoods and possibilities, optimism seems to be the most rational approach. It is certainly the most fruitful and least harmful.

The desire to make whatever life is left pleasing, is what motivates most people. Whether that amount of time is half an hour or twenty years, that usually means leading a normal life. The doctor may have to modify that somewhat with his treatment. But the advice he gives is designed to get the patient back to as nearly his ideal life, with as little disruption as is inevitable, for as long as the most optimistic estimate might allow.

The Therapeutic Value of Optimism

If what you have to tell the patient is encouraging, then saying it is extremely valuable. I once told a patient and his wife that in my opinion he had a normal expectation of life. When he died, only a month or two later, I felt that I would have lost face, but that his best interest had been served by my optimism. I was astounded when the wife wrote and said "You were the only one who gave us hope" and thanked me profusely for it. I realised then that hope is actually better than reality, and that is a thought to bear in mind when discussing a patient's future.

It is perfectly appropriate to be optimistic in the worst circumstances. The disease has happened and nothing can be done now to prevent it. Often nothing could have been done to prevent it at any time. However bad the prognosis, that prognosis is based on average figures, and the patient in front of you may be one of those who does better. In almost every disease which has a bad prognosis there is the occasional patient who seems to be cured, and any patient may be as fortunate. Even incurable diseases have their ups and downs, and the patient who is down should be told that he will be better. The concept of eventual improvement boosts the morale as does the idea that a cure may be round the corner. Finally, and not as rarely as one would wish, the diagnosis may be wrong. For all these reasons the doctor can, and should, take an optimistic attitude and this communicates itself to the patient, with a very positive therapeutic effect.

The value of optimism is not confined to serious disease. If you are forced to advise an unpleasant course of action, it will be more readily acceptable if you emphasise the positive aspects.

Talking to the Patient

As in history-taking, the words you use must be carefully chosen. Technical words and jargon have to be avoided, or when unavoidable, they must be explained. Long or esoteric words and initials are unnecessary and they may be dangerous if they are misunderstood. (A.P. may mean action potential, antero-posterior, artificial pneumothorax or angina pectoris.) The whole aim of giving advice is to be understood by the patient, and anything which impairs that is bad doctoring. If you mumble or speak too rapidly, the patient will not be able to understand what you say.

The doctor who needs a social worker to explain what he really meant is failing in the most important aspect of patient handling. If you lack the insight to see that the patient does not understand, you may need an ancillary worker to tell the patient what you mean. However, the main reason for incomprehension is faulty technique. Sometimes the doctor is so busy that he leaves the explanations to someone else, and this liberates him to perform more intricate tasks. In some situations, and surgery might be one of them, it would clearly result in more patients being processed and shorter waiting lists. But this would be achieved at the expense of proper doctoring. It is a matter of opinion whether it is better to treat two patients moderately well than to treat one patient properly. The answer to waiting lists is to appoint more doctors where that is necessary. Generally, it is only bad doctors who are too busy to finish the job properly. Advice-giving is the climax of patient handling, and it comes best from the doctor who made the decision. The role of ancillary workers should be confined to the innumerable non-medical aspects of the patient's illness. Many patients consult doctors because they want someone to talk to and they may invent a symptom or two to justify the visit. Once you are certain that the symptoms are those of loneliness, a consultation with a nurse or a social worker may be of great benefit.

Talking Down

Patients are drawn from the whole of the population, with its bell-shaped distribution of common-sense and intelligence. It is imperative to adjust your attitude and approach to each individual. This is not "talking down"—which is unacceptable, and which betrays dreadful intellectual snobbery. If you are unfortunate enough to possess this defect you must suppress it in your doctor's role-playing. There is nothing clever about being clever. It comes entirely without any effort on your part and is not correlated at all with niceness or humanity or good citizenship. Knowing all about endocrinology is a badge of knowledge, not a badge of superiority. A patient who is not as bright as you are may be your superior in every other respect. If the patient is a Nobel prize winner in physics, you still have to explain to him the nature of his disease and your reasons for advising the treatment. You have to modify your dissertation "downwards" in a way which would not be necessary if you were treating a colleague.

Although the knowledge flows down the concentration gradient, there is no need to talk down in the patronising sense of those words. You are explaining to a human being what you, in your role as an expert, think he should do. In order to do that you have to use whatever techniques are necessary to get the message across. It is your attitude which makes it appear that you are talking down, not the words you use.

Good Advice, Bad Advising

Some doctors give advice badly, in a way which is upsetting to the patient. There are many reasons for this. If the doctor has feelings of insecurity about his advice to this particular patient, or about life in general, he may compensate by being bossy, or bullying or flippant or hectoring or even by being cruel. All these are attempts at self-aggrandisement in the eyes of patients or colleagues, and although the need for them is understandable, they are self-defeating because in the last resort there is only one way to score, and that is to send the patient out as well doctored as is humanly possible. The doctor must continually be asking himself if he is sacrificing the patient for short-term gains, the net result of which is antitherapeutic.

Tact combined with tactics is the essential ingredient in proper advising. Everything you say must be carefully selected and said with tact. Almost anything can be said in a therapeutic manner if sufficient tact is used. Almost anything may be made frightening and unacceptable if it is inconsiderately said.

Tempo

As consultation has such a disturbing effect on the patient, he should not be given too much advice at one session. He is likely to retain only those parts of the advice which suit him, and it is better to restrict advice at the first interview to essentials, and to repeat a summary of what you said, and extend it, at subsequent consultations.

Monitoring the Reception of Your Advice

As you give your advice, you watch how it is being received and you tailor the extent of your revelations to the patient's expectations and needs. You watch the reception of your every word, and like a driver on a straight road, you make constant fine adjustments of the steering wheel. If you keep the steering wheel fixed, small imperfections in the steering mechanism and the wheels, together with the camber and unevenness of the road, will cause you to end up in the gutter. If you plough on with your set speech, regardless of its reception, it is the patient who ends up in the gutter.

By and large you do make a similar speech each time, because you have the same things to say to patients who have the same disease. Experience teaches you what the "usual" requirements are. If you do this you are less likely to leave something out. But patients vary in the way in which they respond, and you have to make sure that each patient is getting the right treatment, and also that he is being told about it in the way which makes him most contented.

Why a Patient May Not "Hear" When He Listens

A patient may not hear what you say because he has a question to ask which is occupying the front of his mind. Will he be out of hospital by May the 8th which is the day his daughter gets back from abroad? Geoffrey Evans advised us to lower our voice and turn to the students if we had anything we particularly wanted the patient to listen to. Few people can resist listening hard to something they think they ought not to hear. Patients may have reasons for saying that they were not told. If they were not entirely convinced by the first explanation, they may want to hear another doctor's opinion to see if the two coincide. They may not remember exactly what the first doctor said, and would like to hear it again. This is one reason for not giving too long a talk at one session. Most of what you say will be new to the patient and he may not be in the best mood to take it all in, or he may be of limited intelligence. Anxiety may prevent the patient from hearing what you say; Mike Matthews teaches that there is nothing so deafening as a hammering heart. Sometimes a patient says that you haven't told him anything because he finds that what you say is too painful to accept. If he hears it again, he may begin to accept it.

The practice of giving the patient a leaflet about his disease so that he can read what you have said at his leisure sounds reasonable but, like a borrowed suit, it may or may not fit the patient. Leaflets often raise as many queries as they settle. It might seem reasonable to tape what you said to the individual patient and give him a copy. Unfortunately, the presence of a tape recorder is so inhibiting, for both patient and doctor, that the quality of the advice would fall. The patient will "hear" more if your advice is given in the form of a dialogue rather than as a speech.

Showing Concern

Patients watch their doctor for signs that he is worried about them, and such feelings must be suppressed. A doctor may say "I'm worried about..." or "I'm more worried (or concerned) about...," and such phrases are frightening. It is normal to feel concern, but it is unprofessional to show it. The pendulum has swung from the position where the patient was told almost nothing, and sometimes imagined the worst, to the opposite extreme where everyone he meets spends some time "putting him in the picture." This process is just as likely to make him imagine the worst. A friend of mine who had suffered the symptoms of prolapsed intervertebral disc for years was admitted to hospital for investigation. In hospital she revealed that she had difficulty in micturition. When I went to see her, she looked much more worried than she had on admission. "They are all very concerned about my waterworks problem," she said. This level of concern had shifted her view from the hypothesis that "It was only a disc" to "It must be cancer." Fortunately it was only a disc, but demonstrating concern had done her a disservice.

Advice to Children

If the child is old enough and well enough to understand, the doctor should, whenever possible, transact business through the child to the parent, rather than the other way round. Child and parent are told things in terms that the child will understand. If the parent asks a question, the answer is spoken to both of them. Children like to feel that they are the centre of attention and it is just as easy to say to the child "You must..." as it is to say to the parent "He must..." Sometimes the parents try and enlist the doctor's help in order to coerce the child into changing what they regard as a "bad" habit. If it is a non-medical matter, the doctor should not line up with the parents against the child. If it is medical, he should be absolutely certain that the change is necessary, and he should be careful to explain the situation to the child.

The Language Barrier

The difficulties of talking to patients through an interpreter have already been discussed in Chapter 2. Foreigners, even those who speak the language relatively well, may not use words in precisely the same way as the indigenous population. They may convey or receive an impression which was not intended. Patients from abroad often have quite different expectations of their doctor and it may be difficult to determine what exactly they seek. In immigrant families, the men go out to work and learn to speak the language, but the women tend to stay at home with no one to talk to. Deprived of their family support, lonely and unable to communicate even with the sales staff in the shops, it is not surprising that they become depressed and develop symptoms. This possibility should be borne in mind whenever symptoms do not seem to fit into a recognised pattern.

BUILDING UP THE DOCTOR–PATIENT RELATIONSHIP

The Patient's Choice

The patient consults you because you are trained and experienced in treating the symptoms which he has, and about which he is almost always ignorant or ill-informed. Very often he has little choice about whom he consults, certainly not when his general practitioner refers him to a consultant, and indeed very often his choice of a general practitioner is limited. The general practitioner may be the only one in the area, or he may be one of a group of doctors, only some of whom the patient trusts, or he may be a new partner or a replacement of a retired partner in the practice. More and more frequently these days, the general practitioner may be a complete stranger from one of the locum supply services. Even if the patient knows that the doctor has a good reputation, the relationship between a patient and his doctor is a personal matter and they may not suit each other.

Trust

The doctor–patient relationship is based on trust. While you are busily peering at the patient in order to make a diagnosis, he is examining you to see whether he feels that he can trust you enough to take your advice. This trust is not based on an examination of your credentials, although the fact that you are licensed to practise should mean that you have at least the minimum qualifications for the job. The patient's trust is based on the same sort of conclusions as the doctor's advice. He looks at the doctor and decides whether he likes the cut of his jib. He must be convinced that the hair-raising procedure which is being recommended—or even the decision to do nothing—is without doubt the right thing for him in the circumstances. He must go into battle convinced that he is in the best hands.

People are skilled at this sort of rapid assessment, having practised it daily since childhood. Although they make mistakes, some more than others, it is astonishing how right most people are most of the time. Our happiness and well-being depend to a large extent on knowing whom to trust, so we are forced to become proficient.

The Positive Therapeutic Presence

There is a fashion nowadays for honesty in relationships, and this has extended to doctoring. The trendy, ostentatiously not-white-coated physician, who is trying to behave like "one of the boys," may feel that in this man-to-man situation the patient will be happier to take his advice. Whilst there must be some patients who would prefer advice from a "mate," the vast majority like to have their advice from someone who looks as if he knows what he is talking about. This look, like so many other faculties, is partly inherited and partly acquired.

Demeanour is most important. Whilst you are always absolutely serious, there is no place for gravity even if the prognosis is terrible. You may feel that it is dreadful that this twenty-four-year-old woman has a lactating carcinoma of the breast and that she will be dead in a few months. Nevertheless your attitude must speak to the patient reassuringly. If you think to yourself, "Lactating carcinoma. Right. What am I going to do to make the remainder of her life (and it may be much longer than you think) happy and useful?," then your bearing will convey optimism rather than pity.

The Doctor's Image

A great deal of what doctors do depends on illusion. We need it badly because we need to have the patient's trust in order to make him as well as possible. If a doctor is seen walking down the corridor eating an apple, he is probably rushing from a busy morning clinic to a busy afternoon clinic and he is trying not to keep the patients waiting. Even doctors have to eat, and there is nothing shameful or embarrassing or upsetting about the sight of anyone eating an apple while walking. But if a patient thinks that this is surprising in a doctor, then a tiny erosion of his trust takes place. It is irrelevant whether or not the doctor's self-image is dented by what he is doing. When within sight of the patients or their relatives, it is important for him to live up to their image of him because it affects the efficiency of treatment.

A Centre of Excellence

In this chapter I have stressed how inadequate is the basis for your advice, but if you are well trained and a craftsman, it is the best advice which can be obtained in the present state of knowledge. The whole atmosphere in the surgery or in the hospital should give the patient the impression that everything about the place is smart and efficient and that everyone is professional—with all that this implies. An atmosphere like this can be felt, and it gives the patient the confidence he sorely needs. Each doctor should be a personal centre of excellence.

Atmosphere is hard to define and it is the result of dozens of small items of self-control and self-sacrifice on the part of the staff. If the corridors look like the inside of a British Rail train, littered with potato crisp wrappers, cigarette ends and discarded sheets of newspaper, the patient feels that the organisation is run down and inefficient. It does not bode well for the arrival on time of the trains, and it does not bode well for the vastly more important treatment that he is about to receive. Theoretically, there is no reason why the train should be late just because it is dirty. But when an organisation is good, it is usually good from top to bottom, and there is a high probability that slackness in cleaning will be accompanied by slackness in keeping to schedule. Several patients have told me how their spirits rose when they were transferred from a run-down hospital to a centre of excellence.

Ill-considered Advice

Patients understand that treatments change and that if you said five years ago there was no treatment, you may now have some to offer. But if you tell a patient that his symptoms are not sufficiently severe to warrant surgery and then a month or so later, during which time he may have got a little better, you decide that your first estimate was faulty, your change of opinion needs an explanation. Even the explanation that you have been discussing "his case" with your surgical colleague who told you that he is now getting much better results is sufficient to make the patient accept the change of course. If you say one thing, and then say the opposite, the patient is bound to lose confidence. Nothing is gained by admitting that you estimated the situation carelessly or forgot to wait for the result of a crucial test. Craftsmen do not do the job carelessly. If, however, you were in the incubation phase of infectious mononucleosis at the time of your original misjudgement you can undo the harm that would be done to the doctor–patient relationship with a suitable excuse. In proper doctoring the patient must be able to feel that his doctor is competent, consistent and caring. The craftsman aims at impeccable performance from beginning to end with each patient.

"I Had This Myself"

It is generally held, and is I think usually the case, that patients do not like to think that their doctor is susceptible to disease. Thus the effect of telling them that you yourself once had the disease and are now fit and well fails to reassure because you lose your magic. As with most generalisations, there are exceptions and some people are reassured if you tell them. Sick doctors, perhaps because they are fully aware that a medical degree does not confer immunity, seem particularly susceptible to this revelation, and latch onto it with an enthusiasm which indicates that they have temporarily suspended their statistical faculty.

Conflicting Information

Nothing is quite so destructive of confidence as conflicting information. One doctor is in charge of the patient and ideally he should be the common channel for any information. The patient comes into contact with many doctors and ancillary workers, all of whom may offer, or be asked for, their advice. It should be clearly understood who is in charge of the patient. Whilst the doctor in charge must listen to sensible opinions, individual members of the team should be left in no doubt that they are not licensed to give the patient a dissenting opinion or one which conflicts with the party line. There is no place for democracy in giving advice to patients.

If someone says something to the patient which is contrary to the views held by the doctor in charge or says something which should not have been said, then the doctor in charge has to "pull rank." He must say, as tactfully as possible, but with as much authority as is necessary to disabuse the patient, that the information is wrong and that its supplier was in error. It is difficult to say this without loss of face for the culprit, but this is better than loss of the patient's peace of mind. The team member may play an important part in the patient's treatment, so his authority must be left as in tact as possible. He may of course be right and the doctor in charge may know it, but if it should not have been said it must be refuted. This may be a difficult thing to do.

Conscience

A team member may consider that the advice which has been given to a patient is so offensive to his moral principles that he cannot carry it out nor even appear to agree with it. This situation is uncommon, but it does occur. If the team member is quite certain that the matter is a problem of conscience and not merely a difference of opinion, he should thrash the matter out with his chief before he sees the patient.

If discussion does not solve the problem, or if the team member is convinced that his chief's mind has become unbalanced, then he may be forced to resign or to take the matter to a higher authority. Whatever action he decides to take, the differences of opinion should be kept from the patient.

Time and the Doctor–Patient Relationship

In many trades and professions, once you have dealt with an item of business efficiently, you can pass it from your "In" tray to your "Out" tray and forget about it. With patients, responsibility is continuous. If you are off duty or asleep when called, you go and see your patient not because of your innate good nature, but rather because it is implicit in the contract. You do not have guaranteed off duty times, rather you are off duty unless you are needed. When your patient moves to another department, say for investigation or surgery or radiotherapy, you must ensure that the new doctors are informed about any features of your patient's illness which may affect the way in which they handle him. You "hover," if only in spirit, over your patient until he has passed through any difficult period, and you continue to do so after he has left hospital. He remains one of "your patients." Patients usually feel that themselves, and they feel too that although they have been discharged, their doctor would send for them if some successful new treatment was discovered. This is a lofty ideal, but you should aim at it.

The Role of Relatives

Most patients come to consultations unaccompanied, and they may or may not tell their relatives the same story as you have told them. Patients often protect their family from bad news, and the story which the patient tells his relatives is his own concern. As one marriage in three ends in divorce, patient and spouse may be at loggerheads. As the doctor's "contract" is with the patient, he must accept the patient's decision about what the relatives should be told. Of course if this makes treatment more difficult, one can reason with the patient when you are alone together, but the doctor should make every effort to tell the relatives only what the patient wants them to know. The range of information which a patient wishes to keep from relatives is enormous and often unpredictable. A seventy-year-old man asked me not to reveal his true age to his wife; he had added five years to it when they were courting, as she had wanted to marry a man older than herself. He had been living with this "fib" for half a century, and was desperately anxious that she should not find out.

Accepting Presents

Almost everyone enjoys giving and receiving presents. Most patients are worse off than their doctors and you may feel that his need is greater than yours. But the patient who gives you a present has made up his mind to do so, and however large or small it is you should accept it gratefully no matter how you feel about taking it.

HOW MUCH TO TELL THE PATIENT

The Patient's Role in the Decision-Making Process

In an attempt to make medical practice seem more democratic, a great deal of lip service is paid nowadays to the patient's role in the decisions which affect him. In fact the patient's role is limited. The fundamental difficulty is that it is not really possible for the patient to have a worthwhile opinion about the technical aspects of his condition, and these aspects are important in determining what is to be done. There is no way of educating him up to a level whereby he could participate in these aspects, even if he is a doctor in another speciality. It is difficult to put a gastro-enterologist, for example, completely in the picture when he has a cardiac infarction. Although the pros and cons of this or that form of therapy may interest him enormously, he is in no position to choose whether he ought to have it or not. Any pretence of "consultation" on technical matters is bogus. The patient has a number of views about what you propose and he must be encouraged to state them. There may be personal feelings which you have not elicited—for example he may be so frightened of having an operation that he would rather put up with his symptoms than submit to surgery. Sometimes there is a problem of an "administrative" nature; he may be going abroad for six months and would like to get the operation over before he goes, or alternatively he would like to wait until he gets back.

This view of the patient's role is not based on a low estimate of his intelligence. Some patients are more intelligent than their doctor but they know very little about the complicated subject of medicine. When the service engineer tells you that your car needs a new gearbox, you are "entitled" to your view that your car just needs servicing, but you are unlikely to be right. Just as an amiable mechanic will listen to what you say and answer it with a demonstration or an explanation as to why you have got it wrong, so a proper doctor will try to do the same. This is necessary to make the patient content to take your advice, but it is nothing like the democratic process.

Assessing What the Patient Wants to Know

Judging what treatment to advise is the most skilled aspect of medicine. Judging how to advise it is the next. The patient does not have the experience to know how much about his disease he would rather not know. As you cannot know until he finds out, you can have no preconceived notions about "what you always tell patients." Rather, you tell them the minimum amount which will satisfy them and you do not overload them with information that they would rather not have heard. The doctor who always tells patients if they have cancer, or the one who never tells them, are both failing to show the adaptability to the patient which is a hallmark of proper doctoring.

You can tell from experience and insight what patients want to know as you are talking to them. You can tell where they require reassurance, what questions they would like to ask if they dared, what they do not want to be told in any circumstances, and what line to take with them. You must maintain that elasticity of mind which enables you to treat everyone as an individual and to change course when your antennae tell you that your usual line is unprofitable. You must have your answers pat, and it is more important that your story should be consistent, logical and directed towards getting the patient well, than that it should be the whole truth or scientifically accurate.

If the patient decides that he will take your advice, he neither wants you to justify it, nor does he want to hear all the complications, nor does he want a crash course on physiology and disease. He wants to know what you propose to do about it, and in order for him to accept your proposals he has to know a number of things about the situation, which you proceed to tell him. The amount which he wishes to know varies enormously. Many patients brush away even the barest explanation with "I'll do anything you say doctor"; most want an outline description, and a few ply you with questions and then go and read it all up. Assessment of what the patient wants to know is as skilled a process as any other in medicine. Whereas on the one hand, many doctors do not give adequate explanations, on the other, only an articulate minority demands lengthy explanations. The majority of people, often including the articulate minority when it comes to the test, do not actually want to know the details.

At dinner parties, or on TV chat shows, the "advanced" view is that if the speaker had anything wrong with him, he would like to know all about it. A substantial number of the less "advanced" disagree, and they belong to the school of patients who present no problem about how much to tell. The "advanced" people present more of a problem: the question is, how much more do they want to know? I have already said that many healthy people genuinely think that they want to know everything, but that when they are sick, they change their opinion.

The Patient Who Reads a Book About It

There are many popular books written for the layman about living with various diseases, and the point is often made that if you do not tell the patient enough, he will buy a book or look it up in the library. In fact few people do look things up, and even if more did, it would be no indication to tell them all about the disease. The choice of how much a patient should be told should be left to the patient himself. That is to say, as you are giving him your usual, minimal explanation of the disease itself, you look at him to see if this is enough, and you tell him more until he is satisfied. The patient's face exhibits clear signals if he is unsatisfied, or if he does not want to hear any more. These signals, which take time to develop, determine how much you tell, and when you tell it.

A friend of mine was recently discharged from hospital where she was under the care of a well-qualified and well-intentioned doctor. He intercepted her husband and son, whom he had not previously met, as they were on their way to visit her on the day of her admission to the wards and told them that she had cancer of the colon and that it had probably spread to her lungs. The stunned husband, who had been told by their GP that the patient had a urinary infection, asked how sure the doctor was that it had spread to the lungs. He replied that he was 80 per cent sure. The relatives made their way to the ward and could not hide their distress from the patient, who had not been told of the diagnosis. For a week they had to pretend that there was nothing seriously wrong. The doctor then visited the patient and asked her if there were any questions which she would like to ask. She said "No." He asked if she was sure that she had no questions, and she replied "No thank you. I am happy to leave matters entirely in your hands." As the doctor moved to the door he turned and said "Are you quite certain that you have no questions?" She could see that he wanted her to, so she asked if there was bad news. "Yes" he said, "you've got cancer" and then proceeded to tell her all about it in terms which she said were largely incomprehensible.

The patient and her husband and son were a tightly-knit family, and the mother was easily the most sensible, resolute and stable of the three. If—and in my view this was unwise—he felt compelled to reveal the diagnosis, he should have waited until he got to know them before he broke the news. He chose the worst time to tell them, when they were fully occupied in trying to accustom themselves to the fact that the patient was in hospital. In choosing to tell them when they were on their way to see her rather than on their way out, he allowed them no time to master their feelings, and in fact the husband, who was ill-equipped to receive bad news, broke down and cried when he saw her. She could not understand why he was crying, and it upset her.

The revelation that she had cancer was more than enough for a first consultation. If he was only 80 per cent sure that the growth had invaded the lungs, he should have said nothing about that. The patient had only been in the hospital for a day, and further tests showed that the lungs were not affected. He should have waited for all the test results before he gave an opinion with such grave prognostic implications. He delayed for a week before he revealed the diagnosis to the patient, and the husband said that he found it almost intolerable to tell lies to his wife for the first time in their relationship. The patient made it perfectly clear that she did not want to ask any questions and he ignored her signals. His explanation too was incomprehensible.

The family were subjected to a great deal of unnecessary anxiety as a result of this series of misjudgements. They felt that they had no confidence in a man who told them that the lungs were affected, and a day or two later that they were not. It is not surprising that they asked their GP to refer them to someone else.

You may ask the patient if there is anything else he wants to know, and if there is, or if he thinks of a question after he leaves you, your attitude must make it clear that you are willing to answer. Many patients have unforeseeable questions which they fail to ask because they do not want to waste your time. Clearly it is not a waste of time, and is certainly preferable to their worrying about the question until they eventually pluck up the courage to ask. If a patient wants to look it up, that is up to him.

If he does look it up, and asks you about what he has read, you ask him if he can lend you the article. Having read it you can agree with it if you feel that it is true, or does no harm. If in your opinion the article is misleading or wrong, you must say so. If you feel that the effect of the article is harmful, and if you are sure that you will not have to eat your words at a later date, you can say, regardless of whether it is true or not, that the article is not relevant to his case. People are eager to accept the idea that in their own case things are different.

Living by Clichés

Most people lack experience of most of the thousands of incidents which happen in the course of everyday life. For example, many people have no actual experience of anyone close to them dying. If they have, it may not have been the same sort of dying as they are confronted with now. If one of your family is killed outright in a road accident, it offers little or no guidance on how to cope with death from a long-drawn-out and unpleasant illness. And this is true of admission to hospital, or being knocked down by a bus, or being mugged, or even being burgled. The fact that personal experience of these quite commonplace events is so limited, means that we get our "experience" of life largely from hearsay, television, the newspapers, films, the theatre or novels. The doctor must bear this in mind when he talks to patients. He must also bear it in mind when he answers patients' questions. If the patient says "Is it cancer doctor, I would rather know," he may be mouthing the usual cliché which comes out of the mouths of actors when they are playing a sick man. We have a series of conversational gambits which we use in response to bad news. Often the gambit is not meant to be taken seriously, it is simply a way of saying that you acknowledge the news, and will make your dispositions in good time, when you have recovered your balance. Some people who say that they would rather know, have not stopped to consider the implications of knowing. They do not have to consider too deeply to want to know that it is not cancer; that news is always welcome. But if it is cancer, many people close their eyes to the information when it slips out or can be easily obtained. It does seem as if part of the armamentarium of some patients against disease which is likely to be fatal is to pretend that it does not exist.

Auto-suppression of Bad Tidings

The mind is capable of tremendous self-deception. I have known two experienced surgical colleagues of high intelligence who died of cancer. Their minds were perfectly clear when they spoke to me. One said that he clearly would not be ready for work again for a month. The other said that he was so well that he felt that the diagnosis must be wrong. Both were clearly dying at the time they made those remarks, and in fact both died within a month of saying them. Whether they "knew" or not is irrelevant; that is what they said, and it is not the doctor's job to contradict them with the "truth."

This book is not the place for a full discussion on this very difficult matter. I just want to point out that there is a good reason for taking things slowly, and thinking about the true nature of the question before you answer it. At the outset, the patient does not know what he wants to know, and neither do you. You explain as you diagnose, expectantly. You speak when the moment is right and you say what you are certain the treatment demands, or the patient really wants to be told. The important thing is not to say anything which you will be unable to explain or explain away at a later date. Satisfying the patient now, should not be achieved at the expense of a breakdown of the doctor–patient relationship in the future. As in sailing, the aim is to reach the destination, and it is a mistake to lighten ship in a storm by tossing the sails overboard.

The newly qualified doctor may not have the knowledge or confidence to bear the burden of truth on his own shoulders and may off-load it on to the unfortunate patient. Sometimes this behaviour pattern becomes fixed for the rest of his career.

Telling the Patient About the Complications of Treatment

Most patients want to hear that everything is going to be fine, and if it is not going to be like that, you can act therapeutically by concentrating on the positive aspects of therapy. There is no room for gloom or pessimism at the bedside. Anaesthetic deaths do occur, the gas cylinders do sometimes get connected up the wrong way round, wounds get infected, the bones may not unite and some patients are transfused with the wrong blood. All these things, and all the other complications of treatment which have at some time been described, are taken into account before you make your recommendation. Their prevention in the patient under consideration is your problem and that of your colleagues.

It is undoctorly to present the patient with a list of the complications of therapy and ask him to decide whether he is prepared to take the risks. He has no experience of them, and the burden of choice is the doctor's. Once the patient has agreed to accept the treatment which you advise, it is bad doctoring to add to his fears by enumerating more complications than he has already anticipated. The patient seeks your advice on what to do, given the risks of doing it. He is not looking for a menu of complications; he is asking whether you recommend the dish of the day.

The less the patient hears about risk the better, for he has enough on his mind and is busy adopting Nelson techniques for not seeing them. The mind has its own ways of dealing with distasteful matters. It is perfectly reasonable to let the doctor worry about the situation, and to think of something else oneself, and in my opinion this is the ideal situation for the patient. As in talking about investigations, the doctor's reticence about aetiology and prognosis should be balanced by a flood of information about "behavioural" aspects of the disease and its treatment.

Defensive Medicine

There is a school of thought which believes in putting all the complications, no matter how remote, to the patient, either on the grounds that it is only fair, or on the grounds that if the worst happens the patient will have been warned and therefore unable to sue. Patients rarely sue, and when they do it is usually for negligence. The possibility that a conscientious doctor will be sued for failure to reveal a complication is so remote that it should not influence what is said to the patient.

Forewarning

As with investigations, if therapy produces some unpleasant side effect which the patient is unlikely to anticipate, then he should be told about it in advance. For example, if you say that the leg will be sore for a week or so after the operation, because that is where they take the graft from, the patient will then realise that the graft has got to come from somewhere and that you cannot make an incision anywhere without it being sore. So he will not worry when he finds that his leg is bandaged from thigh to ankle, and that it hurts and throbs.

How We Accommodate Risks

We live all the time with risk, such as traffic accidents, and although our attitude is neither calculated nor reasonable, we accommodate to it. In dangerous situations from which there is no escape, or which, like driving a car, cannot be avoided if we are to live a normal life, people adjust to any new risk, and take it in their stride. Many people are sure that they will die under the anaesthetic, and this is a perfectly reasonable fear because they may. Of course if anaesthetic mortality is one in a thousand then one may, but 999 will not. For the one who dies, the mortality is 100 per cent, and unfortunately there is no way of knowing which group you belong to until it is all over. When I visit a patient the night before major surgery, I leave him with the thought that in seven days he will be a new man, or that when he comes round from the anaesthetic he will be free of pain for the first time in ten years. This therapeutic concept provides an antidote to the thought of certain death under anaesthesia.

"Is It Risky Doctor?"

The public has a very poor understanding of statistics and of logic. Since the Second World War, doctors have received a great deal of statistical education which is notably lacking in lawyers and architects and politicians. The patient is unlikely to have a rational approach to the statistics of his situation. Some operations which are familiar to him, like varicose vein or hernia operations, he feels are entirely safe and entirely successful. Other operations, particularly in the thorax or cranium, he regards as very much less successful and more dangerous than they actually are.

Patients occasionally ask if the operation is risky. This question makes me feel that my exposition has failed, for I should have made it clear that the operation was less risky than doing nothing. I suppose some do understand this, but still ask the question, because they had decided to. After all, if you are about to submit yourself to some dangerous procedure, you might reasonably want to know the risk. You might also prefer not to. When I am asked this question, I use a very successful technique which I learned from Wallace Brigden. I ask the patient what risk he would consider reasonable, and invariably the answer is 50–50. Now this is an enormous risk, and almost all the heart operations except transplantation, are done at risks below 10 per cent. The mortality of the safest ones, such as closure of a ductus arteriosus or of an atrial septal defect, is well below 1 per cent.

The practical advantage of asking the patient for his evaluation of the risk is that he is enormously pleased to hear that the risk of dying is 2 per cent rather than 50 per cent. The theoretical interest is that it reveals how wide of the mark the patient's view is and how necessary it is to tell him, whether or not he asks, that the procedure is safe. A homely analogy, like crossing the road, or riding a bicycle in a city, or air travel, or riding a motorcycle, or mountaineering, gives the patient more of an appreciation of the risk than a figure does. Of course the figures of mortality for mountaineering are not available, but it is an estimate of the degree of danger that the patient wants, not an actuarial survey.

What the Patient Does Not Want to Know

Some expressions—enlargement of the heart is one of them— frighten the majority of patients. Before using them, you should estimate whether it is necessary, in the interest of treatment, to tell the patient about the finding. If not, then it is better not to say it. If you are trying to press home the advantages of taking medication for high blood pressure, you can say that the extra load on the heart is reduced by the treatment. It is not necessary to reveal that the heart is hypertrophied or enlarged. It is rarely advantageous to mention a frightening abnormality.

Some patients will already have heard about their "abnormality" before they come and see you. The cardiathoracic ratio measured on a routine chest x-ray may have been greater than one half, and this may have been reported as "the heart is enlarged." The fact that the patient is an athlete, or has failed to take a deep breath, or has such a flat chest that a normal-sized heart is squashed and flattened, may mean that the "enlargement" is not real. This is one of the dangers inherent in the interpretation of tests on their own, out of context of the clinical findings. Lengthy explanation may be required to convince the patient that the finding is erroneous.

If the heart actually is enlarged, but appears to be normal in every other respect, the patient may derive comfort from the concept of the normal distribution curve. As a Parthian shot you can say that his larger than normal heart is no more abnormal than a 6 foot 7 inch man is a giant. If the patient asks you if his heart is enlarged, you should say that there is some enlargement, but never that it is huge, even if the chest x-ray is visible on the viewing box. Patients rarely know how to estimate heart size. The patient whose heart is diseased may regard enlargement as an all or none phenomenon, and the concept that in his case the enlargement is slight, may be therapeutic.

What has been said of the heart is of course applicable to all other abnormal findings.

The Time Element

Time plays an important part in many aspects of handling patients. A difficult diagnosis often becomes clearer with time, either because of some new development, or because the patient lays a different stress on some previously reported aspect. Many difficult problems are solved by taking the history again.

As in dinghy sailing, there is usually only a limited number of courses of action in each situation. It is the timing of these actions which distinguishes the Olympic helmsman from the tyro. The shrewd doctor can sense the slightest change in the wind and bides his time. Time plays a part in the patient's acceptance of his condition. The shock of the news that he is about to lose a limb or one of his faculties, may make him feel that life is not worth living. In time he usually comes to feel that even this great loss leaves a lot of other pleasures.

It is easier to accustom oneself to a gradual onset of symptoms. The patient who is suddenly blinded has much greater difficulty in adjusting than one who loses his sight gradually, not only for the practical reason that he has less time to teach himself to adapt, but equally because the mind accepts anything, given time. Consequently, telling the patient that something awful is inevitable may be better delayed—at least the benefit of delaying should be taken into consideration when the doubt of not knowing is making the patient press for the information.

Time is very important in handling chronic disease. In many diseases the patient may be seeing the same doctor, or his successor, for twenty or thirty years. However long the disease lasts, for the hospital doctor, or for however long the patient remains on his list, from the point of view of the general practitioner, the doctor must be consistent. Your story must hang together. If you adopt a proper paternalistic approach to the patient you will have told him some things and omitted others. You should make a note of what you have told him, so that you do not contradict yourself.

Time and the Patient

Illness has a distorting effect on the patient's sense of time. A man who is willing to queue all night for a ticket to a concert or a football match will often be furious if he is kept waiting when he consults a doctor. Although he knows that it is very difficult to allot appointments because of the unpredictable variation in time taken for consultation, he can see no reason why his appointment should be delayed. Clearly, waiting time should be kept as short as possible, especially for the old, the very young and the frail, who should be seen out of turn if necessary. When patients complain about delay in being seen, I point out to them that there is no way in which a National Health Service can economically offer a service without waiting times. I say that to wait to have a decision about one's health seems to be at least as cost effective a way of spending time as is queueing to see a football match.

One of the advantages of a parallel private system, is that those whose time is enormously valuable, can pay for a service with minimum waiting for about the price of a meal in a good restaurant. This too seems to be a sensible way of spending money.

"They Never Tell You Anything"

Medical students spend a lot of time talking with patients. After years of often boring or irrelevant preclinical work, they are let loose in the wards and they feel that even if they do not know much about examining patients, they can at least talk to them. The patients are a captive audience and they like talking to nice young students who take great interest in what they say, and who can be questioned on aspects of their disease which they are not too clear about. The patients do not realise that the students themselves are not too clear about disease. The students do not realise that talking to patients is an art which is much more difficult than feeling the spleen. Furthermore, the students believe every word the patients say. One invariable result of these conversations is that the students feel that the doctors don't tell the patients anything.

Each generation of students feels this way. I certainly did, but of course in those far off days we were too shy to say anything. The modern student will accost you in the corridor or in the bar and speak his mind. At my hospital we got so fed up with this accusation that we got a pair of students to listen in to the interviews with the patients, and made them record what we said. We sent another pair of students off to see the patients in their homes. Sure enough they came back with the complaint that we hadn't told them anything, but this time we were able to confront them with documentary evidence.

EXPLANATION

The proper doctor maintains an elastic attitude to explanation, giving it as required both for treatment of the patient's disease and for his peace of mind. He is careful about explanations, particularly when all or part of the explanation is speculative, because he may have to eat his words at another time. This is a much more difficult process than saying only what you know to be true in the first place.

Explanation, like everything else the doctor does, is used as a therapeutic weapon, and can be aimed at increasing the patient's motivation towards accepting the treatment. If the patient is given some pills to be taken three times a day, but without any "explanation" of what they are for, he is less likely to remember to take them than if he is told that they will take the load off his heart by reducing his blood pressure. This information, which is so superficial as to barely deserve the name, makes him feel that by taking them, he is helping you to help him. He has a vested interest in getting better, but the explanation makes him a partner in his progress.

The Explanations We Give

Our curious method of making decisions also determines what we say to the patient. As a lot of decision-making is based on guestimates, and other parts of it are the result of sensations which cannot quite be described, explanation is bound to be less than satisfactory. Patients overestimate our knowledge, and the more you tell them about mechanisms, the worse it sounds. Indeed, the longer an explanation is, the more likely is it to reveal its shaky foundations. The shaky foundation is the best we can do at this time. We are steadily improving, and if the patient could wait twenty years we would have a better based medicine. But the patient needs advice now and you give him the best you can, knowing that it is good, but that it will not stand the light of scrutiny.

Inadequate or incomprehensible explanations give no reassurance. The explanation you give should aim at satisfying the patient, so that when you ask him if he has any questions, he says "No thank you Doctor, you have told me all I want to know."

Analogy

The purist frowns on analogies on the grounds that they are rarely exact enough to be accurate. Nevertheless we often think in terms of analogy, and we certainly use analogy to further our understanding of physiological mechanisms. The application of cable theory to nerve conduction has led to a substantial advance in our understanding. In spite of what Richard Asher said about the imperfections of the motor car analogy, the heart for example has much in common with the petrol engine. Many people have a superficial understanding of how a petrol engine works. If you tell them that their problem is something like maladjusted slow running control or a speck of dirt in the carburettor jet, it conjures up a readily understandable and passably accurate image. Many parts of the body have similar mechanical or everyday analogies which are effective in explanation. It is, however, important to make certain that the patient is familiar with the analogy. Most cardiologists understand haemodynamics better than they understand electricity, and they are usually confused when they are offered electrical or mathematical analogues of haemodynamic concepts.

Put a Name on the Diagnosis

It is a surprising fact that many patients do not know the name of the disease for which they are being treated. Whenever possible, the disease should be given a label, and the label should be interpreted where that is necessary. Certain diseases are accepted without explanation by the majority of patients. Stomach ulcers, varicose veins, hernias, piles, lumbago and cancer, hardly require description, although in fact the words cover a range of diagnoses.

If you tell the patient that his symptoms are due to a stomach ulcer, and that you are going to prescribe some pills which will allow the ulcer to heal, you will have told him the diagnosis and what you propose to do about it. If he believes that he knows what an ulcer is, he may not require any further in formation. Alternatively, he may ask why people get ulcers, and how the drug works, etc. He may also wonder, but be frightened of asking, whether the ulcer is malignant. The clinician judges, from the look on the patient's face, if anything needs to be said in reassurance. He may decide on a pre-emptive strike by telling the patient that he has a benign stomach ulcer and that … If the question of malignancy had not entered the patient's mind, it is a pity to put it there by saying that the ulcer is benign.

Once the issue of malignancy is raised, the patient may wonder if the diagnosis that the ulcer is benign is conclusive.

Ill-conceived Explanations

Explanations may backfire. A patient was told that his ulcer was caused by excess acid in the stomach, and that vagotomy prevented the formation of excess acid. When, after the operation, the ulcer recurred, the patient wanted to know how this could be so, as the vagotomy had stopped the excessive acid secretion. The role of acid and the vagus in peptic ulceration is not entirely understood, and it would have been better if the surgeon had simply said that vagotomy allowed the ulcers to heal. Patients understand that in their case the operation has been unsuccessful. But the "pat" story about acid took a good deal of explaining away, and in the treatment of the whole patient it was actually harmful, because the patient became sceptical. The temptation to "clinch" matters by going beyond what is actually known for certain, either about the patient or about the disease process, must be resisted. Patients say, "There must be a cause for my giddy turns." Of course there must be, and there must be a reason why they occur at random times, but although we may be able to find some abnormality of vestibular function, we may never find out why it comes out of a clear blue sky, in a different situation each time. So the "explanation" that it is vestibular is hardly worthy of the name.

REASSURANCE

Most people who consult doctors have no "disease" other than the ageing process, or the symptoms of abuse of their physique. Many other patients have overestimated the implications of their symptoms, so reassurance is one of the main therapeutic weapons, and it may well be the most important. When you have done a particularly good job in reassurance, patients often say "Well, I'm sorry to have wasted your time then doctor." I tell them that far from wasting my time, my favourite medicine is soundly based reassurance. From the point of view of drug kinetics, or of getting your series up to a hundred, reassurance is not as interesting as active therapy, but from the point of view of doing good to the greatest number of people, it is incomparably more effective. In addition, it is going to be your most frequently used therapeutic tool, so you must do it properly, and one of the best ways of doing that is to enjoy doing it. Train yourself to derive more satisfaction from reassuring patients than from giving them drugs. Unlike so many drugs, it actually does the patients good.

All illness leads to anxiety, even when that anxiety is not expressed. You should ask yourself what fears are engendered by the disease which the patient has, and you should give the necessary reassurance.

The Misuse of Drugs

William Evans used to teach that reassurance is the most precious pill which we administer. Many patients do not require any other medicine, but the "busy" practitioner often "saves time" by prescribing drugs which alter mood, in what he takes to be the appropriate direction. He then spends a great deal more time administering other drugs to counteract the side effects of the "mood benders," and the patient is no better for any of the medicines. When the patient can be satisfied with a verbal explanation, it is malpractice to administer drugs. William Evans coined the aphorism "It is better to do nothing than something, when nothing needs to be done." Dornhorst made the same point with his inversion!" "Don't just do something, stand there!"

Patients with organic disease are often—and entirely reasonably—depressed by their condition. If they are reassured about its nature, they rarely need antidepressant drugs, which anyway seem to be largely ineffective when used to suppress appropriate, unreassured, inadequately explained anxiety. The idea that an organ, though diseased, has untapped functional reserves, is more antidepressant than any pill.

Practical Aspects of Reassurance

Reassurance begins during the history-taking. The way you react to the patient's symptoms can be reassuring or terrifying. So too in the physical examination, your mien reassures. If you take a history which is absolutely diagnostic but which the patient feels has been too short, it will impair the efficacy of your reassurance at the end of the interview.

In the physical examination your response to the findings with raised eyebrows, cluckings and cries of unbelief, will be fertiliser to the seeds of fear which the symptoms have sown. Again, if the examination appears to be too short, the patient will feel that you could easily have missed some important sign. A skilled craftsman can examine a system extremely quickly. Complete examination of the heart, extracting every physical sign, can be done in less than two minutes, and a speedy neurologist can examine that system in three minutes. In an emergency, one often only wants to know one sign before taking action, and this may only take seconds. If the history is not that of organic disease, it is important to take an adequate amount of time in examination, particularly of the part which is giving rise to the symptoms. "He didn't even look at it" precludes successful reassurance. Certain investigations have a magical significance to the patient. The electrocardiogram, whose contribution to the health of nations is slight, is one. If it is normal, or said to be normal, it has a profoundly reassuring effect, in spite of the fact that a significant number of patients with ischaemic heart disease have a normal graph. This should not deter the clinician from using a normal graph as a weapon to "prove" that the patient has a normal heart.

Equivocal Test Results

In most tests there is an overlap between normality and abnormality. If the doctor decides that the patient is normal, he must ignore the equivocal results and put the abnormal ones to the back of his mind. Your reassurance must be wholehearted even though your information is frequently incomplete. If you based everything you said on the most cautious or the most truthful statement, you could never reassure anybody about anything. If the patient is normal, much harm can come from telling him about equivocal or "false positive" results. If the patient has already been told of the result, or if there is a likelihood that the test will be done again at a later date, the clinician must explain to the patient that tests are fallible, and that in his case the test is wrong. The patient must be told that if the test is done again the result should be ignored. A great deal of harm is done if unconvincing or half-hearted reassurance is given. In neurotic patients symptoms are like forest fires: the earlier and more firmly they are stamped out, the less likely are they to take over. The more neurotic the patient, the more reassurance he needs.

Reassurance Without Strings

William Evans taught of the importance of not qualifying reassurance. If the patient is entirely normal, then no qualification is necessary. If however he has some disease, some qualification may be necessary. A patient whose ruptured Achilles tendon has been successfully repaired may ask if he can play games. If the tendon ruptured while playing football, it would perhaps be stupid to play again. But if the man was a professional or had a good chance of achieving some lifelong ambition in the game, he might be prepared to risk its going again. He may not realise that a second repair will be made more difficult by the first operation. If you put the "cost" clearly to him, he may make his own decision. This is not the sort of string that William Evans was referring to. He was referring to the reassurance that the pain was not coming from the heart, followed by advice not to hurry, just in case the pain was atypical angina, that dreadful ragbag of doctors' indecisiveness.

The way you put your "string" matters enormously. If a patient asks you if he can go back to playing football, you can point out that he is at the age when most men give up rough games; if you add that he could play tennis, or golf, or sail or swim or ride, your string will lose much of its sting.

The Technique of Reassurance

Reassurance takes time. "It's nothing to worry about" or "You're normal," although pleasing to hear, is not an effective therapeutic dose. Having clearly given the matter enough thought, and the patient enough examination and tests, you sit him down comfortably, look him in the eye and looking pleased you say "I am pleased to tell you that the symptoms which you describe are not those of…The examination was absolutely normal, and so were the special tests that have been done. You have a normal.…" You do not say that you could not find any abnormalities, because this might mean that they escaped you because you were not looking in the right place. It might also mean that although the organ in question was diseased, your examination and tests were not sensitive enough to detect it. This of course is always possible, and it is one of the places where a test can be so useful. If it is non-invasive, or requires only minimal assault, it may be used as a weapon to "prove" that there is no abnormality, and that the reassurance is soundly based. A surfeit of tests is unreassuring, but if the patient is suitably primed beforehand, by "I am sure that your… is normal but this test will tell us for certain," then a test may be therapeutic for those who appear unwilling to accept a clinical estimation.

Some patients prefer instant reassurance, and if the doctor's certainty is totally convincing, they accept it delightedly and rush away before you can suggest a test or two. Others need two or three repetitions of a message of reassurance, dotting the *i*'s and crossing the *t*'s, before they can accept it. You have to make up your mind during the consultation which type of person you are dealing with.

"I Would Like to See You Again"

If you are quite sure that the patient is normal, your reassurance is undermined if you ask him to come and see you again about that particular problem "just to be on the safe side." If you find a shadow in his chest x-ray which is almost certainly "inactive," you are forced to re-examine his radiograph after an interval. You can say that you are sure that the x-ray change is of no significance but to make assurance doubly sure, your routine is to re-examine in three months. If you add that you are sure it will be normal when you do it again, you mitigate even if you cannot eradicate his anxiety.

The Advantage of Being an Older Doctor

Age is an advantage in giving an opinion of any sort, particularly in giving reassurance. It is easier to believe the reassurance from a grey-haired doctor than it is to take exactly the same words from a youth half your own age who looks as if he is too young to know much about it. William Evans says "Age buys experience, and in medicine, experience is a precious commodity."

Some years ago I developed symptoms and signs of carcinoma of the rectum. I consulted a wise physician who listened to my textbook story and asked a number of questions. When he had finished taking the history and before he had examined me, he said that this story was not that of carcinoma of the rectum. I found this statement totally convincing, and although he went on to examine me, and order the appropriate tests, his *ex cathedra* statement had already cured me. He had spent years listening to such stories and, like other experts, he could tell that what appeared to a cardiologist to be classical, was in fact a fake.

"What Causes the Pain Then?"

If you tell the patient that his symptoms have no organic basis, he may find it difficult to accept that the sensations he experiences, which he didn't previously have, can have "no cause." This is particularly the case if the symptoms have a sudden onset. When the doctor says that there is no organic abnormality and that the symptoms are functional, the statement covers a range of aetiology from deliberate invention to symptoms which are outside the patient's control, as for example hiccoughs, cramps or extrasystoles. Although these symptoms must have a cause, we commonly do not know what it is, and there are no pathological changes which we recognise. The symptoms will not "harm" the patient in that they do not alter his expectation of life nor his power to enjoy it. This latter is not a very sharp endpoint, and is to a large extent a matter of opinion. Headaches are a good example. Almost everyone has the occasional headache, and that cannot be regarded as a disease. If, however, the same mechanism causes daily or weekly headaches, it may be disturbing enough to rank as a disease.

Headache is a useful example to give to patients with other symptoms. They can accept that the pain that they get in the chest or in the abdomen is analogous to the occasional headache. This implies that it is real and not due to neurosis or imagination, but that it is not a cause for alarm and that the mechanism is not known for certain. The occasional headache is one of the few "functional" symptoms that almost everyone can accept without demur. Patients do not like the concept that the symptom is imaginary or the result of neurosis, and in fact it is much more commonly the result of minor abuses of the body. People expect a headache if they take too much alcohol, or pain in the legs after unaccustomed running or horse riding, and most functional symptoms are due to this sort of abuse, or to bad habits. Faulty chewing or posture, overeating, straining at stool, irregular bowel habits, or mechanically inappropriate ways of carrying things, together with the disuse atrophy of chronically under-used muscles, are the causes of most function disorders which do not have an obvious, pathological basis.

Another class of disease which might reasonably be included in the category of "functional" are the diseases of excessive response to internal or external stimuli. Asthma, migraine, vaso-vagal attacks and palpitation often have no "cause" which can be identified, save that they are precipitated by factors which do not cause those symptoms in "normal" people. In some cases we can demonstrate that the mechanism concerned, although normal from the anatomical point of view, is unduly responsive, and then the disorder of function itself can be considered as a disease. These disorders of function are so common that they do not carry the stigma in the patient's mind which other functional symptoms carry. It is a pity that these different sorts of functional ailments are not given different names.

Symptoms Which Occur at Random Times

Some patients with symptoms which occur in paroxysms ask why the attacks come out of the blue, at random times. The answer that they are precipitated by independent circadian variations in one or more of his biochemical systems which summate to produce a stimulus which triggers an unusually sensitive end-organ, never seems to give much satisfaction even when it is translated into English. The mechanism of such paroxysms is fascinating to both doctor and patient, and many patients spend a great deal of time speculating, and altering their way of life to avert the attacks. In most cases they are forced to the conclusion that the attacks are random; in my experience the "explanation" that "it is just one of those things" seems to be as acceptable as the biochemical one.

Minor Disease

Both functional and organic disease may be minor in degree. The patient may have symptoms which are not sufficiently troublesome to warrant treatment. A firm diagnosis may be impossible without a number of investigations which may involve risk or discomfort which is out of proportion to the severity of the symptoms. After appropriate examination, the mature clinician will not be ashamed to tell the patient that he does not know what the diagnosis is, but that he is sure that it is not serious and will not shorten his life nor affect its quality enough to warrant investigation or treatment. I learned from Mike Matthews that such patients are helped to accept the symptoms if you explain that the brain acts as an "editor." When asked, it will tell you that there is a pressure of clothes upon your shoulder, but normally these signals are "edited out." Similarly an alerted brain will "edit in" and give undue amplification to a minor signal.

Risks to Relatives

The relatives of patients with serious diseases are often unduly worried that they too may have the disease, and the patients themselves wonder whether they may transmit the disease to their offspring. In some diseases where chromosomal abnormalities occur, the inheritance probabilities have been fully worked out and in these diseases professional genetic counselling is helpful. In the other congenital abnormalities or diseases which have some tendency to run in families, the patient should be told that although the risk is higher than for the average person, it is still extremely small. Some patients come from families with strong histories of diseases like perforating peptic ulcer or cardiac infarction. It is worthwhile pointing out to these patients that, as so many factors are involved in producing the disease, their chance of having inherited it is no greater than their chance of exact physical resemblance to their parents and siblings.

Reassurance of Unspoken Fears

Patients often have fears about the implications of their symptoms which take the doctor by surprise until he has some experience.

These fears often originate from "folklore" and many of them were once grounded in fact, but therapeutic advances have made them no longer justifiable. Haemoptysis, which used to mean consumption and death, is still disproportionately worrying, even though the modern treatment of tuberculosis is effective, and usually requires no change in the way of life. Tinnitus makes people fear that it is caused by a neoplasm; palpitation gives rise to thoughts of sudden death; arthritis conjures up the phrase "crippled with...." People think that if shingles meets in the middle of the body, the patient will die. All these fears and many more have to be brought out into the open. In Dr. J. N. Blau's memorable phrase, the physician must "Ferret out the fear," and the patient has to be disabused of his belief. Once that is achieved, the symptom itself seems to lessen in intensity. A patient who has been unable to sleep because of tinnitus finds that following examination and proper reassurance that it is not due to a cerebral neoplasm, his insomnia goes.

Follow-up

Two different objectives are served by follow-up. The first is that the reassurance that the follow-up visit gives contributes to the treatment; secondly it enables the clinician to assess the patient's progress. Patients should not be seen too frequently because it makes them think that they are more ill than they actually are. Over-attendance may induce a feeling of dependence on the doctor which is inappropriate to the severity of the illness. The doctor's time is better spent on those patients who need him. The date of the follow-up visit is determined by the nature of the disease, and if you decide that you should see the patient in three months, it is quite useful to ask yourself whether it would make any difference to the patient if you had decided on four months instead. If not, opt for the later date. Whenever possible, the time between successive consultations should be increased, because patients deduce from this that they are making satisfactory progress. The clinician should make it quite clear whether or not he wishes to see the patient again, and if not, he should give his reasons.

The second objective of follow-up is to educate the clinician. Follow-up serves to evaluate diagnosis, judgement and therapy, and to teach the natural history of disease. Theoretically all patients should be seen again at intervals even if the clinician is sure that they are normal, but this would overload the clinic and would impair the efficacy of reassurance and induce neurosis. In practice, the element of self-education should be taken into account when deciding on the timing of the next visit. To achieve both of these objectives, it is important to find out why a patient has failed to keep a follow-up appointment, and whenever possible, to induce him to make another.

HELPING THE PATIENT TO ADJUST TO THE FACTS

Patients get relief from the concept that their condition is common, and when their disease is serious, they are relieved to hear that it is not only common, but easily treated or not a threat to life. They are delighted to hear that in their case the disease is "slight" or "mild" and has a better than average prognosis. If the disease is mutilating, or has a poor prognosis, there is almost always some well-known person who has gone on to live a full life after such an illness, and you should quote these people to the patient. Whenever possible you should arrange for the patient to talk to someone who is successfully coping with the same disease. This is enormously encouraging, and is one of the strengths of the Patients' Associations. If a disease is limiting, like angina, patients may find it more acceptable if they think of it as a nuisance rather than as a threat, and they find consolation in the concept that "worse things happen at sea." Patients who were previously extremely fit and have had little or no experience of disease resent the fact that their body "has let them down," and need more reassurance than those who are used to illness.

"You Will Have to Learn to Live with It"

This hackneyed expression gives rise to a great deal of unhappiness. Although the doctor may be advising adaptation, patients usually think that he means acceptance. People adjust to most disabilities, so adaptation rather than acceptance should be the keynote of your advice. The doctor may be able to help with advice and the patient should be encouraged to devise his own adaptations.

"There Is Nothing More We Can Do for You"

This dreadful expression conjures up visions of the home for incurables in the patient's mind. The doctor usually means that there are no more medicines or special measures which will help the patient, or which are necessary or justifiable. This is a faulty estimate of the situation, because there is always reassurance, re-education, encouragement and adaptation. Even on the rare occasions when the estimate is accurate, the words themselves should be avoided. Rather, the patient who knows that he has a serious disease should be told that whatever difficulties arise, there will always be ways of helping. People associate disease with pain, and they are greatly relieved to hear that in their case, pain is unlikely. If it is likely, they are pleased to hear that it can and will be relieved.

Advice Which Is Hard to Take

If a patient is to lose a limb or an organ, or is to have a serious operation, he will be more willing to accept that it has to be done if it is clear that everything else has been tried and has failed. If the symptoms are unpleasant, he will regard it with less horror than would a symptom-free person. The words a doctor uses to convey bad news are enormously important. If you say "I'm afraid that we have got to remove that leg" it sounds entirely negative. If you say "You would be better off without that leg" in a tone of voice which is considered, unequivocal, and indicates that you realise what this means to him, you plant a seed of hope that, in spite of the loss, his life will be better. There has to be appropriate bereavement for the loss of a limb, but hope is powerful displacement therapy. The patient may not know that one can lead a normal life without a kidney or a spleen or a lung, and he will be delighted to hear that one can. Colin Milburn played cricket for his county after losing an eye, and this information is as encouraging to the patient who is about to have an enucleation as it must be perplexing to the vision physiologists.

The Therapeutic Value of Praise

If a patient has done anything to help himself, particularly something which requires self-discipline, you should congratulate him. Even when the patient has played no role in his treatment, he will be delighted if you tell him how well he has done, and will proudly tell his family what you said.

Retirement

It was formerly held that retirement should be put off at almost any cost because lack of occupation led to boredom and death. Whilst this may be true of work addicts, the health of many patients is dramatically improved when they give up boring, stressful or demanding jobs. This is particularly the case if they have other interests to cultivate.

IF THE PATIENT REJECTS YOUR ADVICE

You give the patient the advice which in your opinion will best suit him and it is his right to refuse that advice. His reasons for rejecting that advice must be examined with the same care that you gave to your diagnosis. So you must ask him what they are, before you show the slightest reaction. If his reasons are irrational, your response will depend on how important it is that he takes your advice. You should never be disapproving or exasperated, even though you have made a great effort, and spent a great deal of time thinking about him—time which is actually "wasted" because you could have devoted it to thinking about other patients. You "owe" the patient your full involvement from the moment he consults you, but he does not owe you his compliance with your advice. You may think he is foolish and you may be right. But you may also be wrong. Medical fashions are transitory, and doctors differ widely in their treatment of the same condition; when you compound that with the poor basic foundations on which your advice is based, its rejection should strike you as not at all surprising. Many doctors, knowing the poor quality of their advice, nevertheless get angry when it is rejected. This is bad doctoring. Acceptance or rejection of your advice should be taken in the same unemotional way.

A proper doctor never rejects a patient, although it is quite possible to ask a colleague to take over the treatment of a patient who is not benefiting from your advice, just as a physician would ask a surgical colleague to operate.

Don't Coerce Him, Convince Him

If the patient has varicose veins and refuses your advice to have them ligated, there is little in the way of harm or danger in leaving them as they are. If he goes on to get ulcers, they may prove refractory to treatment, even if he then has the veins tied. The existence and the incidence of such a complication, which is the hidden cost to the patient of ignoring your advice, must be made clear, but the risk of complications should not be used to coerce him. If, however, failure to treat now is certain or very likely to be harmful to the patient, you try to convince him to change his mind, not portentously and threateningly or admonishingly, but as one human being to another. You have your informed opinion, he has his views; is there any way of bringing the two together?

If you handle patients properly from the outset, your advice is unlikely to be rejected. You should regard rejection of your advice as a professional failure, and you should ask yourself where you slipped up. In your zeal to maintain a low failure rate, you may press too hard on the patient. This is always unsatisfactory: firstly because you are taking unfair advantage of him, secondly, because a patient must enter into the spirit of the therapy with enthusiasm if he is to derive full benefit from it, and thirdly because if the treatment is unsuccessful, both you and the patient will regret your having pushed him into it. You give advice unequivocally and firmly.

If you omitted to tell the patient at the outset that you give patients the same advice as you give to your family, you can tell him that when you sense that he may be going to reject the advice. You repeat the reasons for your advice, and stress the advantage of compliance. If you offer him time to think it over, you will avoid an outright rejection, which makes the patient feel that he has offended you. Some patients do not like being told what to do, and if you give them time, you give them the feeling that they are accepting your advice rather than your orders. Many doctors treat non-compliant patients as though they were intellectually subnormal children or ill-behaved pets. Just as a dog's owner is the main determinant of its behaviour, so it is often the doctor's fault if the patient will not take his advice.

Why Your Advice May Be Rejected

Sensible patients may be overawed enough to take silly advice for a short period, but in the long term they are only prepared to take advice which seems to be appropriate. Though they know little about medicine, they have an innate sense of "making the punishment fit the crime." If you tell a patient who has very little wrong with him that unless he goes to bed for six months you will not answer for the consequences, you may frighten him into bed. But after a day or two he will be up and about his business. Advice may not be taken because it does not suit the individual patient. Other patients appear to take the advice but do not act on it. Advice must be tailored to the individual patient. There is no point in giving advice which the patient is incapable of carrying out or unwilling to comply with. A patient may accept the fact that being overweight puts more strain on an arthritic knee joint, and that if he lost weight he would get less pain. But eating may be his greatest pleasure in life, and he may prefer to keep the pain rather than give up his favourite foods. Alternatively, he may not have enough self-control to diet.

Some patients reject advice because they have heard that the drug which you are prescribing is dangerous or has some untoward side effect. If this is the case and they tell you about it, you may have to work very hard to displace erroneous information, or to persuade them that the risk is worth taking. The patient may not understand the risk he runs in not taking the medicine, and he should be told that you prescribed it after having weighed up the risks and the advantages.

A patient may stop taking a drug because he knows that it is poisoning him. It pays to take notice of the patient's intuitions in these matters. Non-compliance is the doctor's best safeguard against appearance in the coroner's court.

Advice Involving Self-control

It does seem odd that a patient who actually takes the trouble to come and consult you and who decides that he trusts you enough to take your advice, should then need motivating if he is to keep on taking it. Man is not gifted at self-control and he has great difficulty in disciplining himself to do anything which he does not particularly want to do. This is especially true if it is long term or not enjoyable. The popularity of self-discipline has declined, and this has therapeutic implications. Persistence with treatment, perhaps for a whole lifetime, may require a good deal of self-discipline from people who have neither the training, the inclination nor the experience to exhibit it. If one is encouraged from birth to be self-indulgent, it is extraordinarily difficult to switch on self-control, particularly if one is being asked to give up something enjoyable. If a patient eats like a pig, smokes like a chimney or drinks like a fish, he may well be recommended to give up one or all of these habits. The doctor must be authoritative if this advice is to be taken and it is very doubtful if his authority is sufficient to make the patient give up the habits of a lifetime. It is even more difficult if the doctor is overweight, smells of whisky and has nicotine-stained fingers.

Overweight

Many of my patients are overweight, and I give them a long talk about what can be summed up as "power to weight ratios," and a diet sheet. If they fail to respond, I step up my talk to the "every pound you lose gives you an extra year of life" story. I gradually harden up my advice, through several more visits, until I reach the "digging your grave with your teeth" homily. Occasionally, obsessional patients strip off the weight with a remarkable effect on their symptoms and their well-being. But the majority stay about the same, and quite a substantial number actually put on weight. This experience is common, and addiction to food or alcohol or tobacco or idleness is difficult to treat. If you watch a patient as you urge him to exercise self-restraint you may see his face harden. This usually indicates that he is not going to take your advice.

Enlisting the Relatives' Help

Sometimes you can "use" the relatives in the patient's best interest. If the spouse is present when the patient is given advice which calls for sustained self-discipline, it makes it more difficult for the patient to ignore it. If the spouse knows that the patient is to lose weight, or eat less salt, or take more or less exercise, or not climb ladders, the patient has to run the gauntlet of the spouse's disapproval as well as his own conscience. This of course runs counter to my previous statement that the patient must be free to take your advice or leave it. Medicine, like life, is a matter of compromises, and it is not possible to practise good medicine without an element of paternalism or enlightened, well-intentioned persuasion.

Fringe Medicine

One characteristic that all unorthodox forms of medicine have in common is that their claims to effectiveness have never been subjected to scientific evaluation. Enthusiasts for the methods, whether it be the suitability of whole foods for the whole man, or "nature's way" or the wisdom of the East, accept their chosen method for reasons which do not seem to be adequate to the impartial observer. Many of the claims do seem to be ridiculous, but some could be real. It is likely, for example, that a pharmacology based on Eastern plants will have some medicaments which are as potent as morphine but which Western physicians have failed to take up. Similarly, the environment and way of life are now acknowledged to play a role in the aetiology of disease which would have been denied only fifty years ago. Our ignorance of aetiology and therapy should condition our reception of unorthodox ideas; they should be given proper consideration. A balance must be struck, for although it may be true that if the patient had led a different life more in accordance with "nature" he might have escaped his present illness, it is also true that now he has become ill, the clinician's concern is to get him better. One may argue whether a neoplasm is due to nature or nurture, but it is certainly more "natural" than the surgery which will cure it. Nature does not always know best.

Evaluating Unorthodox Advice

It is a mistake to belittle other sources of information, unless they are harmful, and you have to consider very carefully what is harmful and what is not. If the patient has been told that some diet or harmless preparation will do him good, it is therapeutic to say that it can do no harm. One should not fail to take advantage of a placebo effect simply because it is unorthodox, or because someone else thought of it. The profession is generally thought to be too orthodox, and patients like to think that their own doctor is broadminded enough to give serious consideration to anything which might be beneficial. One can never be certain that diet or strange herbal remedies will not be effective; food allergies cause many symptoms, and morphine, digitalis and quinine are herbal remedies. The main danger of ineffective remedies is that they may put off the time when the patient seeks effective remedies. A school-friend of mine "treated" his haemoptysis for four months by smoking herbal cigarettes. So if your advice is sought about fringe medication, you must ensure that proper medication is taken too, if it is required.

DRUGS

Drugs come quite a long way down the list of the priorities in treatment. Therapy is traditionally stratified as rest, diet, hygiene (now rechristened lifestyle) and only then drugs, followed by special measures such as surgery. A large number, if not a majority of symptoms can be cured by attention to the first three categories alone.

Taking Pills Is Tiresome

Taking pills is boring; it imposes a discipline which the patient may resent, and as soon as he starts to feel a little better he tends to stop taking them. There is also the feeling that in taking pills, he is "sick" and not "healthy." Taking pills is a constant reminder of mortality. The curious effect of disease on the mind has already been discussed in the chapter on history-taking, and it is no less evident when it comes to taking advice. In spite of the fact that the unpleasant symptoms are responding to therapy, without producing any side effect, some patients will stop taking the tablets. One or two of my patients have seemed to become fed up with taking pills, have stopped doing it, and died as a result; they seemed to me to know what they were doing. This book is not a suitable place for going into all the reasons for failure to comply with easy instructions, but they are manifold and the clinician has to take action against them.

Failure to take the medicines is much commoner than doctors realise, and if there is a failure of therapy, the patient should be closely questioned about the details of his drug regimen. Whenever possible drug levels in blood or urine or stool should be measured. Sometimes the tablets are being taken, but they are not absorbed. The ranges of bodyweight, degree of absorption, sensitivity to and excretion of drugs are astonishingly wide, and must be called into question if the patient fails to respond. The patient is titrated against drugs, using symptoms and signs as an indicator. Frequently, the "usual dose" is too small or too large.

Promoting Compliance

Prophylaxis against non-compliance includes adequate explanation and motivation. The patient should be left in no doubt about the advantages of compliance. Further aids are simple instructions, giving the smallest number of different pills at regular intervals and, once therapy is established, reducing the number of pills by using combination tablets wherever that is possible. The doctor's interest in the medication improves compliance, and each time the patient is seen he should be asked about his medication, and about side effects.

Most drugs produce side effects, and when these are unpleasant, changes should be made in the timing or dosage of the medicaments in an attempt to palliate them. When alternative therapy is available, this should be substituted. The appearance of side effects puts another weight in the balance against treatment, and this new situation has to be reweighed.

As the patient recovers, and his symptoms disappear, the side effects loom larger than they did when he was ill. Getting up at night to pass urine is a joy when you know that it is a manifestation of the process which will cure your orthopnoea, but it is a nuisance if you are sleeping well. Whereas it may have been necessary to administer "round the clock" therapy when the patient was ill, this should be discontinued as soon as possible. Preoccupation with side effects, particularly if they are trivial, should be welcomed as a sign that the patient is getting better.

Groups like Alcoholics Anonymous, Weight Watchers, anti-smoking groups and exercise clubs can often maintain motivation by making people compete against each other, and also by giving support to each other.

Stopping Drugs

Drugs which are no longer needed should be stopped. Sometimes the doctor is uncertain whether the symptoms will recur or not if a drug is stopped. If the symptoms are serious it is best to err on the safe side, and keep the patient on the drug, especially if there are no untoward side effects. If the recurrence of symptoms is without danger, it might be reasonable to reduce the dose or stop the medicine, keeping a close eye on the patient in case the symptoms recur.

Extremist Attitudes to Drugs

Most people take a reasonable attitude towards drugs, realising that they are an integral part of treatment and that they vary from the innocuous to the dangerously potent. Two extreme views are met with, and the clinician must be ready to counter them.

As a result of the thalidomide disaster both the public and the medical and nursing professions have been made over-conscious of the side effects of drugs. Moribund patients are denied heroin because of the risk of addiction, and this very human overswing is responsible for a great deal of unnecessary pain and suffering. A patient may ask you if there are side effects to a drug or risks to a treatment. If you tell him that doing something and doing nothing both carry a risk and that the basis for your advice to him is that the risks of the treatment are less than the risks of doing nothing, that will almost always be enough. The realisation that all medicaments which are effective may produce adverse reactions has only just begun to be accepted by the general public, and this has led to an over-reaction against them. Some patients point out unequivocally that they "don't like drugs," and I tell them that I share this dislike.

Whilst one must guard against therapeutic nihilism, it is a mistake to prescribe any drug unless the advantages of taking it outweigh the risk, and only after the preceding elements of therapy have failed to relieve the symptoms. Drugs and other forms of active therapy are the last resort. If you explain this, most patients will understand that the disease process has resisted the *vis medicatrix naturae*, and that pills are necessary. It is best not to refer to medicines as drugs, because to many people the term connotes addictive drugs.

Some patients are so anxious about pills that this impairs the efficiency of the drugs which they are given. This effect varies with the drug. It is unlikely that the effect of antibiotics will be impaired if the patient is anxious. But drugs which work on hormones or on those organs which are affected by the patient's psychological state, for example the alimentary system, the cardiovascular system and the nervous system, may lose some of their efficacy if the patient is obsessed by side effects.

Doctors too have been over-influenced by the publicity of side effects, and many patients are given inadequate dosage of drugs.

Doctors who are over-influenced by fear of side effects give medicines without enthusiasm. The patient can see that the doctor is not entirely happy about the drug and he starts therapy without the positive placebo effect and with the anxieties mentioned above. When the drug is new, or is the subject of a clinical trial, the doctor's reservations, warnings and lack of enthusiasm prejudice the effectiveness of the drug. Drugs should be presented with enthusiasm; "This medicine is very effective in this condition" or some such introduction initiates a cure before the patient has taken the first pill.

This form of introduction helps to counter the other form of extremism about drugs. Patients sometimes say "He only gave me some pills," and this feeling may date from the days before the Second World War when so few medicaments were effective. The patient should be told that we now have very powerful drugs which are effective.

Drug Interaction

Whereas one should always be on the look out for interactions, one should not be unduly influenced by theoretical drug actions. "If we are already blocking sodium entry with drug A, adding drug B, which blocks calcium entry, will cause ..." Our knowledge of the mechanism of drug action is so primitive that the postulated results rarely occur, and they should not stop us giving an additional drug where that drug is thought to be of value.

Warning About Side Effects

Some drugs—and the contraceptive pill is one of them—are issued with a list of side effects and dangers which is antitherapeutic. In the case of the contraceptive pill no mention is made of the incidence of each complication, so the list of disasters which may occur serves only to haunt the more sensitive user. With drugs which are designed to cure, the patient should be warned of those side effects and any likely side or toxic effects which may have to be accepted or which may be countered by a reduction of the dose. If disturbing side effects occur and the patient has not been warned, he may decide not to take the drug and it may be impossible to persuade him to restart. In order to avoid this situation and to reduce the incidence of such side effects, initial dosage should, whenever conditions permit, always be small. The patient may be disappointed if this does not prove effective. He should be told that because the effective dose in any individual is unpredictable and because it is always better to take as little as is needed, you always start treatment with a small dose and that failure to respond to this may only mean that the dose has to be increased. It is my practice not to tell a patient about toxic effects which are rare or which he will not sense himself. If the drug may produce a leucopenia, then it is the clinician's job to test for it, and nothing whatsoever is gained by telling the patient about the possibility, which had already been taken into account when the decision to administer the drug was reached.

Almost everyone realises that an overdose of most drugs will cause symptoms, and the patient will not be made apprehensive if you tell him that the dose for the individual patient is difficult to forecast and if you tell him what action to take if one of these symptoms develops.

Failure to Respond to a Drug

The other side of the coin is that one is frequently asked to see patients who have "failed to respond to . . . ," and one finds that for reasons of weight, absorption, distribution, excretion or sensitivity, the usual dose was for them inadequate. The dose of a medicine of choice should be increased from the minimum effective level to the maximum tolerable level before the drug is abandoned as being ineffective. The recommended dose is usually the average dose, rather than the largest amount which may be given safely.

In those situations where the drug chosen stands quite a high chance of being ineffective or badly tolerated the patient should be told that there are many different drugs for his condition, and that it may be necessary to try several before one is found which suits him.

Dispensing Errors

A patient may fail to respond to treatment or describe unusual side effects because he has been given the wrong drug. Pharmacists as a profession are remarkably efficient and rarely make mistakes. Indeed they are trained to check up on the prescriptions which they dispense. Dispensing errors may occur because the names of drugs are sometimes similar enough to be confused with each other. For example, chlorothiazide the diuretic, may be confused with chlormethiezole the hypnotic and anticonvulsant, especially when the handwriting is bad. Geoffrey Evans used to say "If you want your name to be well known, write it so people can read it" and he used to advise us to write legibly or print the names of drugs. As in the above example, it may be better to use the proprietary name (Saluric) if you are too busy to print the name.

FATAL DISEASES AND DEATH

"Putting His Affairs in Order"

A prevalent fallacy among both doctors and patients is that people ought to be told that they are going to die if only to "put their affairs in order." This concept has a pretty, archaic ring about it, but does not stand up to examination. Most deaths are the result of cardiovascular disease or accident and hence most people die suddenly, without any forewarning. These people obviously do not have time to put their affairs in order. As sudden death is common, most men and women of affairs already have them in order. Little is gained by changing the handling you have decided on, in order to forewarn a patient, except the off-loading of responsibility. Many people cannot bring themselves to put their affairs in order for one reason or another. If the patient dies intestate, it does make more trouble for his family, but once again the patient's interests take first place. He may want to spend part of his last days making arrangements for the distribution of his possessions, but he may not. In practical terms there are very few affairs of sufficient importance to the dying to make it worth while upsetting their last days.

The Patient with an Unfulfilled Ambition

Occasionally someone who has a limited future uses the time to do something which he has always had an ambition to do, but which he has put off for one practical reason or another. Theoretically, the knowledge that it is "now or never" very occasionally means that the patient would rather know the prognosis in order to be able to carry out his plan. This situation is extremely rare. Although one should bear it in mind, and respond to it if one knows it to be the case, it should not colour one's advice to patients too much.

What to Tell the Relatives

At the other extreme a patient with a fatal disease may not want his family to know that he is soon to die, either because he does not want to upset them, or because he cannot bear the effect this will have on their attitude towards him. One of the worst aspects of disease is other people's solicitude. Their constant enquiries, fussing and covert glances to see if death is imminent, and their sorrow and pity, may be harder to bear than the disease itself. It is quite impossible to lead a normal life—which is the stated aim—if you become the target for all this unwanted attention. The patient may be sensible and balanced and the spouse may be unstable, so what you tell such a spouse should be guided by what the patient thinks would be suitable.

Sometimes relatives come and speak to the doctor or phone him up and ask questions. The doctor should bear in mind that what he says may find its way back to the patient. In their intense desire to do something for the patient, relatives sometimes blurt out "Well the doctor said . . . ," and the patient will recognise that the doctor did not say that while the relative was present. An erosion of confidence results when this happens. As such revelations are common, the doctor should not say anything to the relatives which the patient must not hear. It is best to tell the relatives only those things which the patient already knows. The doctor should tell the relatives that he will inform the patient of their conversation. If the relatives misquote the doctor to the patient, he may ask the doctor about it. If you have already told him about the talks with, or the calls from, the relatives, you can explain that they must have misunderstood what you told them at that time. If he challenges you, and you have not told him of the conversations, you then have to admit to private talks with the relatives. Your confession undermines your power base, and he wonders how much more there is to find out about your faithlessness.

Many patients, though, lean on their close family who give splendid support, and in these conditions the family may want to know things which the patient has not thought about, or which he has not been told. Once again, you must not satisfy the relatives at the patient's expense. The contract between you and the patient is valid until he is dead. What you tell the relatives must be governed by the knowledge that what you say is very likely to get back to the patient. A secret is defined as something you tell nobody. Sometimes a change in the relatives' manner will allow the patient to detect that some information has leaked.

Off-loading a Sense of Failure

A doctor may find relief in telling the relatives that the patient is doomed, as a result of an incurable disease. This excuses the failure to cure which, in the present over-expectant atmosphere, may have made the doctor feel that his performance is not up to standard. Incurable diseases present a challenge to the doctor but he must beware of either "trying anything" to show that he has left no stone unturned, or unloading his feelings of failure onto the patient or his relatives. The doctor's task is to do everything that can be done, and not things that can't. A good deal can be done to alleviate the physical and psychological effects of incurable disease and the anguish of relatives.

Leaving No Stone Unturned

Relatives whose concern for the patient may have been shamefully inadequate during life, sometimes try and make up for twenty years of neglect by a last-minute endeavour. They may also put pressure on the doctor to do more tests and seek other opinions "to see if anything can be done." Most doctors are optimists and they may succumb to the desire to try anything. It is difficult to resist this temptation, but the principle to bear in mind is that the patient should not be made to suffer to provide a clear conscience for the doctor or the relatives. The threshold of pain or discomfort is low in the elderly and infirm. Even a vital capacity breath may give rise to a sore chest.

Forewarned Is Forearmed

Unexpected bereavement upsets the relatives, and they suffer less if they know in advance that the patient is going to die. Most people can see when a patient is deteriorating and the knowledge that he will die dawns on them gradually. This is preferable to the shock of being told. Some people have false hope which prevents them from seeing what is inevitable, and then and for other material reasons they may have to be told. The patient's interests still come first, though, and duty to relatives is secondary.

A relative has to be told even more gently than the patient, because it is often easier to bear the thought of your own death than the death of someone you love. Furthermore, the patient may have had intimations of his death from the symptoms, and may even be glad that he is going to be free of them. The relatives have no such advance warning or compensation. Relatives should be given as much help as is possible, because they need it, and provided that the patient's interests are kept in the forefront, little harm will be done. Serious disease may have a profound psychological effect on the relatives, and allowance must be made if they behave abnormally.

Fatal Diseases in Children

As with adults, the inaccuracy of prognosis and the small gain from pessimism means that the sensible doctor will be optimistic and will try to make whatever time the child has left as pleasant as possible. If you have made it clear to the parents that the disease will prove fatal, they are likely to ask how long you estimate the child will live. If you say that survival time is very variable and that "it could be years" and then say that we must all see that the years are as full and normal as possible, the relatives will derive satisfaction and hope.

The Hospice Movement

In any one year, only about eight or nine patients on the "list" of a busy general practitioner will die. Most of these will die suddenly from vascular disease or accidents, and only one or two patients per annum will die in a way which demands long-term attention from the practitioner. In hospital practice too, such deaths are rarer than one would expect. The result of this is that few clinicians have enough experience of the varied aspects of terminal care to be able to ensure that the patient has a dignified death and that pain is controlled and consciousness is clear. Many problems, both in drug therapy and general management, arise in this situation. The available drugs are so different in their actions and in their suitability for the individual patient, that terminal care has become another speciality, like ophthalmology or radiotherapy, in which the generalist is unlikely to be competent.

Most doctors have accepted this situation, particularly once they have seen a patient who was confused and still in pain, transformed in twenty-four hours to become pain free and clear-minded. Some doctors nevertheless feel that they are best able to carry out terminal care. In the case of exceptionally gifted or well-trained clinicians, it is true that the doctor who has handled the patient from the beginning will know him best and will—other things being equal—be able to handle him best. Unfortunately, other things rarely are equal and some clinicians, in my opinion wrongly, feel that they are threatened by the implication that specialist help is needed. If terminal care units could be seen in the same light as are paediatric units, that is to say they are called in, without loss of face, by all sorts of other clinicians when they need help, the patients and their relatives would benefit.

The Role of Religion in Terminal Care

Another great advantage that these units have is that they are often run by people with strong religious convictions. Many doctors do not possess these convictions, and thus they lose the assurance which most religions give, and which believers are able to transmit, that life is only a prelude to some better form of existence. I find it extremely difficult to regard death as anything but the end of everything, and this is an impediment when dealing with the dying, who are often more willing to believe in a hereafter when they are near death. I have observed agnostic patients, to whom I had been unable to give adequate comfort, dying almost joyfully after a conversation with a colleague who had strong convictions about life after death.

An agnostic can of course reassure a dying patient about the "course well run" if he knows enough about the patient. In practice one rarely knows how satisfying someone else's life has been and even when one does, it can hardly offer the same sort of consolation as does religion.

Talking About Death

Many doctors are embarrassed when talking about death to patients and it has been referred to as the last remaining taboo. The doctor may feel that if he knew more, the patient might not be dying, and this adds to his discomfiture. However, if the patient wants to talk about death it is wrong to deny him this opportunity. Of course the things which one can say about it are limited to the mechanics of the situation, but it is usually this aspect which the patient most wants to discuss. Patients frequently worry that death will be painful, and they need reassurance that it is usually not painful, and that any pain which may occur will be relieved.

8. ATTITUDE TO COLLEAGUES

HEARSAY

Our Gang

People who have some characteristic in common feel more secure if they band together, and they derive innocent, if not very sophisticated fun from deriding anyone who is outside the group. This schoolboy humour must not be allowed to spread to the consulting room. "Well, you know what surgeons are like" may evoke contented smiles at the Physicians' Committee, but it will chill the blood of a patient who is about to be operated on.

"Dr. So-and-So Said . . ."

A patient may tell you about advice which he has received from another doctor which seems to you to be irrational, useless or dangerous. Never be tempted to say "That never works" or "That might easily give you kidney failure." Sometimes the patient will tell you that his disease was diagnosed in terms which have now become unfashionable. "Tired heart" and "weak lungs," once respectable, now raise a laugh. The doctor may have had reasons for doing or saying what he did, or he may have been silly, or the patient may have misreported him. Whatever the origin of the offending statement, nothing is gained by deprecating comment. Patients often remain intensely loyal to doctors who have failed them, and they rightly suspect your motives if you allow surprise, shock or incredulity to influence your comments.

Your own sense of insecurity is what usually provokes adverse comments; as everyone except a manic depressive in the manic phase of his illness has such feelings, you must learn to live with them, and not try to assuage them at the expense of your relationship with the patient. The most effective balm for insecurity is immaculate performance.

"Who Did That to You?"

You should also refrain from comment on what appear to be incompetent operations by other people. Although you must ask what the operation was done for, it is a mistake to say "My goodness, what a horrible scar" or "Who on earth did that to you" or, worse still, "That looks like one of Mr. So-and-So's operations." The patient has to live with the scar, and if he thinks that you, as a doctor, are shocked by it, he will assume that laymen will be even more disturbed when they see it. One never knows the difficulties under which the surgeon was working, nor what damage had been done by disease before he operated. Infection quite outside a surgeon's control may play havoc with the neatest of scars, as can keloid. Even if the scar is the result of incompetence, nothing is gained by comment, and the professional approach is to keep your opinion to yourself.

Critical Comment by the Patient

Sometimes a patient will make denigratory remarks about a doctor he has seen in the past. It is necessary to have a stance to deal with such remarks. The doctor may or may not have done something silly or thoughtless or wrongheaded, but in his absence there is very little likelihood of getting at the facts, or at what was in his mind at the time. Discussion of the matter is therefore a waste of time, and it offends against the elementary concepts of justice, in that one is "trying" a man without giving him an opportunity to defend himself. If you defend the doctor, you weaken the bond between you and the patient, and the patient will discount what you say on the grounds that "they always stick together."

If what the patient says is clearly untrue, you may be tempted to say "I don't believe he said that." This too is antitherapeutic, because it can only mean that you are saying that the patient is not telling the truth. I have on occasion heard a patient say such awful things about his former doctor that I have felt it incumbent upon myself to make some comment if only to stop the patient from saying it again. In this situation I tell the patient that it is unfair to say damaging things, whether they are true or not, about a person who is not there to defend himself. I try to convey by my manner that I do not want to hear tales about colleagues, because they are irrelevant to what the patient came to consult me about, and that I am not prepared to adjudicate between him and his former doctor unless I can hear both sides of the case in full. I suspend judgement, and I hurry on to another subject as quickly as possible.

A Response to Conflicting Advice

When you have given a patient an explanation and your advice, he may say "Why then did Dr. So-and-So tell me to do . . . ?" The answer may be that Dr. So-and-So is a fool and idle to boot, but he may have been misreported, or he may have given what appeared to him to be the best advice at the time. Whilst you do not cast doubt on the patient's version of events, you say that the previous doctor would have given the advice which seemed best at that time. You may add that it is quite likely that at the time when that advice was given, the disease was in an earlier, and less obvious state of its development. If that argument is untenable, you can say that there are many ways of treating the same disease, some of which appear to be incompatible with each other. Again, I try and give the impression that delving into the past without the evidence serves only to divert our attention from the matter which concerns both of us at the present.

Giving Evidence Against Colleagues

A doctor who is asked to give evidence against a colleague is faced with a conflict of interests. As a just man he will want to see that justice is done to his patient, and I have already commented on how easily any patient becomes "my patient" as soon as you are enlisted in his aid. He will also, if he is normal, often feel that but for "the grace of God" he might easily have been in either the patient's or the colleague's shoes. When the colleague's failure is serious, it is wrong to identify with him. It may be true that "It could have happened to anybody," but quite often a more accurate appraisal is "It could have happened to anybody who was careless or incompetent." The fear that you too may be careless or incompetent at some time cannot be used to excuse an incident which has damaged a patient.

It is in the interest of the profession that negligence should be paid for, and in my view it is not paid for often enough or adequately. At the same time, many opinions which are expressed seem to be unduly biased in favour of "my patient," and whilst I do not advocate a "cover up," it is important to be absolutely just when making assertions about a colleague's performance, and to limit them to the known facts.

SECOND OPINIONS

When Required by the Doctor

General practitioners, especially those in group practice, commonly ask advice from a partner or from consultants. No one is expected to know everything, and no loss of face is involved in seeking advice. Similarly in hospital practice, a great deal of use is made of second opinions, and often third or fourth opinions too. The more specialised you are, the easier it is to seek a second opinion. Sometimes a general physician or surgeon, especially one with an interest in some other speciality, who feels that his general competence may be called into question if he asks advice, is slower to ask for a second opinion, and may wait too long. The more confidence you have in your own ability, the easier it is to ask for help. The patient must not be made to pay for the doctor's insecurity, and you must school yourself to ask for a second opinion when you or your patient need one.

When Required by the Patient

In view of the high stakes involved, and of the difficulty in assessing the skill of one's doctor, it is surprising that so few people ask for a second opinion. Patients generally ask for a second opinion only when they are unhappy with some aspect of the way in which the first doctor has handled their illness.

Geoffrey Evans always welcomed a request for a second opinion, on the grounds that if the second opinion was any good, he was bound to confirm the Evans view, and that the consultation would serve as a subtle way of advertising just how good that view was. Clearly, if the patient is unhappy it puts everyone's mind at rest if he sees another doctor, and the wise clinician will almost always agree to such a request. Many doctors lack Evans' securely based self-confidence, and if such a doctor feels that a second opinion is not necessary, he may have to grit his teeth before he accedes to the request. For the patient is saying that he does not have enough confidence in you to take your advice. At best, such an opinion is unflattering, but as you know that you have made mistakes in the past, you cannot be sure that this patient will not be the next entry in your mistakes book. It may be difficult for you to accept such a reflection on your competence, particularly because it is unusual for a patient to question one's judgement. A good doctor is always questioning his own judgement, but that is not the same thing. It is, however, almost always a mistake to refuse a second opinion, because the patient will remain unsatisfied, and you should train yourself to appear to welcome the suggestion.

Choosing a Second Opinion

A second opinion should be a good one and should be someone who the patient will find congenial. Whenever possible, he should be seen to be independent. Sometimes the patient will name the doctor he wants as a second opinion. In either case, the referring doctor is free to make it clear, in advance, if he disapproves of the second opinion, and he is free to accept or reject any new advice which may be given. If he rejects it, it should be rejected gracefully, and no pressure should be put on the patient.

The Consultation

The clinician who comes as a second opinion should know why his help is needed before he sees the patient. His approach may well be modified by this knowledge. The reason for the request is usually implicit. If for example a general practitioner or a physician asks a surgeon to see a patient with an inguinal hernia, he is asking whether the surgeon would take over the management of this aspect of the patient's treatment. If the referring doctor has any information which might alter that management, then the surgeon should be told about it in advance.

If the second opinion is being asked because there is uncertainty about the diagnosis or the treatment, this too should be made clear, and often there is no intention to hand over the management to the second opinion. Again, the second opinion should be told in advance about the nature of the problem, and what role he is expected to play in its management. This enables him to present the patient with the combined view of his medical advisers. He can say "Your doctor and I think..." without any need for consultation. When the situation does demand further discussion, this should take place in the patient's presence unless it is thought that the patient might be disturbed by it. Whenever the situation is not straightforward, the referring clinician should, if possible, be present at the consultation. If the second opinion has been requested by the patient, it is usually better if the referring physician is absent, because his presence might intimidate the patient.

If the second opinion agrees about the management of the patient, the patient should be told. If he disagrees, then he should say that he will discuss the problem with the referring clinician, and that they will then come and talk to the patient about their proposals. If the second opinion agrees with what has been done, he should lose no opportunity to boost the patient's faith in his own doctor. If he disagrees, he should do as little harm as is possible to that relationship.

The Patient Who Leaves You for Someone Else

If as a result of consulting a second opinion, or for any other reason, a patient decides that he no longer wishes to be under your care, you must ensure that there is no change in your attitude towards him, and if you meet by chance, it is therapeutic to enquire about his health.

"What Are Your Views On...?"

Many people have an inexhaustible curiosity about medicine, and you will often be asked for your opinion. Quite often doctors in other specialities will ask for your opinion, and one should tread warily. In a proportion of cases, the doctor is asking advice about himself, and he will not take into account the fact that you are unacquainted with the details of his condition, and can therefore only give a broad and misleading, average picture.

You may be asked your opinion of other doctors, and it is wisest to be circumspect, and whenever you can, approving, for the questioner is frequently under the care of the doctor he is asking about.

COLLEAGUES AS PATIENTS

It is very flattering if a colleague of whom you have a high opinion consults you about his own health. It is sometimes said that you should not treat friends or relations because your judgement is impaired by emotion. Geoffrey Evans on the other hand took the view that colleagues and friends deserved the best possible advice, and so he had no alternative but to treat them himself. For most of us, this would mean passing the colleague over to someone else.

The philosophy that you treat your patients as you would your close relatives, should ensure that in most cases you are prepared to treat your colleagues without any deviation from your usual practice, and with the same confidence. It is essential not to change by one jot your method of taking a history, routine of examination or ordering of special tests. If you take a short cut, or omit, on "humanitarian" grounds, a test which you would normally do, you are courting disaster. The reason you have the tests done on your "ordinary" patients is because they are necessary, and I cannot think of any circumstance in which a test becomes unnecessary because the patient is a doctor.

When he is ill, a doctor's behaviour is likely to be quite as irrational as a layman's. You may not have to explain that the bile duct drains into the duodenum, but you do have to make your plan of campaign absolutely clear to him, and you must take care to be specific about the details of what he must or must not do. The general tenor of your attitude towards his treatment should differ very little from your attitude to the treatment of patients who are not medically qualified. In general sick doctors are more apprehensive about the nature of their condition, but they are more easily reassured than laymen.

RELATIONS WITH NON-MEDICAL COLLEAGUES

Every year the number of doctors who work entirely alone diminishes. From the general practitioner with his receptionist to the army of non-medical staff in hospital, most clinicians work in association with others. The "chain of command" is of necessity pliable. The most exalted clinician who "orders" sleeping tablets for one of "his" patients would be distressed if the humblest nursing probationer did not "disobey" his "order" if she found that the patient was already asleep when she went to administer the tablets. He would expect her to keep her eye on the patient and give the tablet if she judged the period of sleep to be too short. Administrators, ambulance men, nurses, pharmacists, physiotherapists, radiographers, scientists, social workers, technicians and a host of others—named in alphabetical order rather than in order of responsibilities—all work on the premise that they must use their own judgement when carrying out those duties which they have been asked to do.

As everyone, doctors included, is normally distributed for judgement it is clear that the "wrong" decision will be made from time to time. Although the patient is under the nominal care of a particular doctor, he is also under the care of everyone else who makes a decision about him and under the overall "care" of the Health Authority too. Allocation of responsibility is important from the medico-legal point of view, but it is not germane to the everyday running of a health service. Whether he is legally responsible or not, or whether he is "in charge" or not, the clinician must feel responsible for everything that happens to a patient under his care. At the same time he must recognise the element of autonomy in the role of all the other workers in the service, and he must acknowledge by his manner, and as often as possible in words, that they do an essential job, to professional standards. People work better if they are asked rather than ordered to do things, and they thrive on respect. Most often, the desire to do the job properly is enough to ensure that decisions are taken in a reasonable way, and if the course followed is not exactly as had been envisaged, it is at least an alternative which does not adversely affect the patient.

When the patient is made to suffer, then the mechanism by which the mistake occurred must be sought out as calmly and neutrally as possible. This is best done in private conversation rather than at open meetings. When someone has done his best he has the right to have his mistakes pointed out in private. Such "inquests" should never be held in the patient's hearing, because it would undermine his confidence. If someone persistently does not do his best, or if that best is not good enough, man to man discussions may not be sufficient to improve matters. In these circumstances the best course is to talk to the miscreant's superior; it is almost always a mistake to reprove him yourself.

It seems to me that one of the "perks" of working in a health service in which almost everyone is underpaid, is that when sick, all co-workers should be given a prompt and efficient service, the excellence of which makes it clear that their efforts are recognised and appreciated.

ENVOI

THE PRACTICE of medicine has changed dramatically during my professional lifetime. The difference is due in part to developments in our understanding of the scientific basis of the subject, but this factor has not been as remarkable or as affecting as the change in attitude to disease and to treatment.

When I was a student, most illness was thought to be due to "an act of God." We recognised a few "acts of man"—the industrial diseases for example—but it was thought that the majority of diseases struck like lightning, at random. Another difference in our attribution of cause was our attitude to psychosomatic disease. Only a handful of diseases were thought to be caused or modified by the patient's mind. A third difference was that "positive health" was regarded as the concern of a small number of doctors who specialised in what was then known as Public Health. They were mainly concerned with sanitation and the working conditions in factories. Few doctors felt that they had a role to play in keeping the nation healthy; neither did the public. Most of us felt that our role was analogous, albeit at a higher level, to that of a garage mechanic. We were concerned with repair rather than with design or misuse.

The smaller number of tests then available were more often used to establish the diagnosis than to exclude disease. The reverse is now true.

We used to offer treatment in a different way. Whereas the best doctors have always explained what they were doing, given reasons for their decisions, and encouraged the patients to take the medicines, the average doctor would hand out therapy much in the way a postman delivers letters. That is to say, he is required to deliver them, but not to ensure that you read them. The view was that the patient consulted a doctor because he wanted to be rid of disease, and that the doctor's job was to give him something which would achieve that end. Once the patient had been given the prescription or the advice on a take it or leave it basis, it was assumed that he would take it, and that the doctor's task ended there. He would of course try again if the patient failed to respond to treatment. The patients' expectations were low and they did not seem to find the *de haut en bas* ethos offensive. I am glad to say that they now do—undue humility is hard to take—and this change in demand has been a major stimulus to better performance.

THE RESPONSE TO CHANGE

The information explosion can be coped with relatively easily if you read the journals, listen to your colleagues and keep an open mind—not too open a mind because that may allow the best things to fall out, and they may be replaced with misconceptions. You must find a filter of the correct mesh which governs the flow into and out of your mind. If you change your routine with every innovation, you will not be able to assess your results properly. Good clinical practice needs a relatively stable data base.

The change in attitude to psychosomatic disease has inverted the previous situation and it is now felt that there are few diseases which are not either wholly or partially influenced by the mind, both in their genesis and in their cure.

At the turn of the century the expectation of life of a neonate was 50 years. It has now increased to 73 years. It is argued that this improvement is due to social conditions rather than to medicine, and I am quite certain that this view is wrong. However, regardless of the cause, the fact is that people are living longer and they have been relieved of the burden of infectious diseases and a host of other illnesses which formerly killed many people in middle life. As serious disease has become less common, so patients have begun to take their lesser symptoms more seriously. This means that doctors are consulted earlier, and on more "trivial" matters. Triviality lies in the eye of the beholder, but the trend has necessitated a change in the doctor's view as to what is trivial and what is not; a good working rule is that a patient is unlikely to come to see a doctor unless there is something which is troubling him, but of course the presenting symptom may not be the real reason for the visit. There can be few people who enjoy the inconvenience of coming to see a doctor. The spirit of the times has necessitated a great change in the way in which we view our role. So much for change.

UNCHANGING ASPECTS

Many of the attributes of a proper doctor remain unchanged. The first consideration was, and remains, common-sense. Like height, it is largely genetically determined. As it is difficult to define, and even more difficult to measure, it is not possible to tell whether it can be changed or not. I fear not. The next most important attribute of the effective clinician is his professionalism. This means taking a personal pride in getting everything right every time. One of the most harmful sayings in the language is "Everyone makes mistakes." They do, but what distinguishes the craftsman from the botcher is that he takes care to make as few mistakes as possible. This difference in attitude makes a world of difference to the incidence of mistakes. As Shakespeare says, "lay not that flattering unction to thy soul." You must act on the assumption that by taking care you can avoid making any mistakes.

The open-mindedness which characterises your attitude to information is absent from your attitude to your professional principles.

You practise within a rigid self-imposed framework. Although you are in theory prepared to change a principle, you rarely do. You may change one as an act of will if after prolonged consideration it no longer seems to be correct, but you do not allow your principles to slide for an instant. If for example you have a rule that you never subject a patient to a test that you would not have yourself in like circumstances, then you stick to it all times.

The last of the many characteristics of the complete clinician which I mentioned in the first chapter, and the one with which I would like to end the book, is the concept of your role. You have your job simply and solely to "service" the patients. That is what you are trained and paid to do. You are "In service." This does not imply that you are servile, but it means that whilst you have an interesting, rewarding job and are paid reasonably well, your main function is to satisfy the needs of the patients. It might be worth reading the passage below the book's dedication again.

SUBJECT INDEX

TITLES IN SERIES

For a complete list of titles, visit www.nyrb.com or write to:
Catalog Requests, NYRB, 435 Hudson Street, New York, NY 10014

J.R. ACKERLEY Hindoo Holiday*
J.R. ACKERLEY My Dog Tulip*
J.R. ACKERLEY My Father and Myself*
J.R. ACKERLEY We Think the World of You*
HENRY ADAMS The Jeffersonian Transformation
RENATA ADLER Pitch Dark*
RENATA ADLER Speedboat*
CÉLESTE ALBARET Monsieur Proust
DANTE ALIGHIERI The Inferno
DANTE ALIGHIERI The New Life
KINGSLEY AMIS The Alteration*
KINGSLEY AMIS The Green Man*
KINGSLEY AMIS Lucky Jim*
KINGSLEY AMIS The Old Devils*
WILLIAM ATTAWAY Blood on the Forge
W.H. AUDEN (EDITOR) The Living Thoughts of Kierkegaard
W.H. AUDEN W.H. Auden's Book of Light Verse
ERICH AUERBACH Dante: Poet of the Secular World
DOROTHY BAKER Cassandra at the Wedding*
DOROTHY BAKER Young Man with a Horn*
J.A. BAKER The Peregrine
HONORÉ DE BALZAC The Unknown Masterpiece *and* Gambara*
MAX BEERBOHM Seven Men
STEPHEN BENATAR Wish Her Safe at Home*
FRANS G. BENGTSSON The Long Ships*
ALEXANDER BERKMAN Prison Memoirs of an Anarchist
GEORGES BERNANOS Mouchette
ADOLFO BIOY CASARES Asleep in the Sun
ADOLFO BIOY CASARES The Invention of Morel
CAROLINE BLACKWOOD Corrigan*
CAROLINE BLACKWOOD Great Granny Webster*
NICOLAS BOUVIER The Way of the World
MALCOLM BRALY On the Yard*
MILLEN BRAND The Outward Room*
SIR THOMAS BROWNE Religio Medici *and* Urne-Buriall*
JOHN HORNE BURNS The Gallery
ROBERT BURTON The Anatomy of Melancholy
CAMARA LAYE The Radiance of the King
GIROLAMO CARDANO The Book of My Life
DON CARPENTER Hard Rain Falling*
J.L. CARR A Month in the Country*
BLAISE CENDRARS Moravagine
EILEEN CHANG Love in a Fallen City
UPAMANYU CHATTERJEE English, August: An Indian Story
NIRAD C. CHAUDHURI The Autobiography of an Unknown Indian
ANTON CHEKHOV Peasants and Other Stories
RICHARD COBB Paris and Elsewhere
COLETTE The Pure and the Impure
JOHN COLLIER Fancies and Goodnights

* *Also available as an electronic book.*

YASHAR KEMAL They Burn the Thistles
MURRAY KEMPTON Part of Our Time: Some Ruins and Monuments of the Thirties*
RAYMOND KENNEDY Ride a Cockhorse*
DAVID KIDD Peking Story*
ROBERT KIRK The Secret Commonwealth of Elves, Fauns, and Fairies
ARUN KOLATKAR Jejuri
DEZSŐ KOSZTOLÁNYI Skylark*
TÉTÉ-MICHEL KPOMASSIE An African in Greenland
GYULA KRÚDY The Adventures of Sindbad*
GYULA KRÚDY Sunflower*
SIGIZMUND KRZHIZHANOVSKY The Letter Killers Club*
SIGIZMUND KRZHIZHANOVSKY Memories of the Future
GERT LEDIG The Stalin Front*
MARGARET LEECH Reveille in Washington: 1860–1865*
PATRICK LEIGH FERMOR Between the Woods and the Water*
PATRICK LEIGH FERMOR Mani: Travels in the Southern Peloponnese*
PATRICK LEIGH FERMOR Roumeli: Travels in Northern Greece*
PATRICK LEIGH FERMOR A Time of Gifts*
PATRICK LEIGH FERMOR A Time to Keep Silence*
PATRICK LEIGH FERMOR The Traveller's Tree*
D.B. WYNDHAM LEWIS AND CHARLES LEE (EDITORS) The Stuffed Owl
SIMON LEYS The Hall of Uselessness: Collected Essays
GEORG CHRISTOPH LICHTENBERG The Waste Books
JAKOV LIND Soul of Wood and Other Stories
H.P. LOVECRAFT AND OTHERS The Colour Out of Space
DWIGHT MACDONALD Masscult and Midcult: Essays Against the American Grain*
NORMAN MAILER Miami and the Siege of Chicago*
JANET MALCOLM In the Freud Archives
JEAN-PATRICK MANCHETTE Fatale*
OSIP MANDELSTAM The Selected Poems of Osip Mandelstam
OLIVIA MANNING Fortunes of War: The Balkan Trilogy*
OLIVIA MANNING School for Love*
JAMES VANCE MARSHALL Walkabout*
GUY DE MAUPASSANT Afloat
GUY DE MAUPASSANT Alien Hearts*
JAMES MCCOURT Mawrdew Czgowchwz*
WILLIAM MCPHERSON Testing the Current*
DAVID MENDEL Proper Doctoring: A Book for Patients and Their Doctors*
HENRI MICHAUX Miserable Miracle
JESSICA MITFORD Hons and Rebels
JESSICA MITFORD Poison Penmanship*
NANCY MITFORD Frederick the Great*
NANCY MITFORD Madame de Pompadour*
NANCY MITFORD The Sun King*
NANCY MITFORD Voltaire in Love*
HENRY DE MONTHERLANT Chaos and Night
BRIAN MOORE The Lonely Passion of Judith Hearne*
BRIAN MOORE The Mangan Inheritance*
ALBERTO MORAVIA Boredom*
ALBERTO MORAVIA Contempt*
JAN MORRIS Conundrum*
JAN MORRIS Hav*
PENELOPE MORTIMER The Pumpkin Eater*

ÁLVARO MUTIS The Adventures and Misadventures of Maqroll
L.H. MYERS The Root and the Flower*
NESCIO Amsterdam Stories*
DARCY O'BRIEN A Way of Life, Like Any Other
YURI OLESHA Envy*
IONA AND PETER OPIE The Lore and Language of Schoolchildren
IRIS OWENS After Claude*
RUSSELL PAGE The Education of a Gardener
ALEXANDROS PAPADIAMANTIS The Murderess
BORIS PASTERNAK, MARINA TSVETAYEVA, AND RAINER MARIA RILKE Letters, Summer 1926
CESARE PAVESE The Moon and the Bonfires
CESARE PAVESE The Selected Works of Cesare Pavese
LUIGI PIRANDELLO The Late Mattia Pascal
ANDREY PLATONOV The Foundation Pit
ANDREY PLATONOV Happy Moscow
ANDREY PLATONOV Soul and Other Stories
J.F. POWERS Morte d'Urban*
J.F. POWERS The Stories of J.F. Powers*
J.F. POWERS Wheat That Springeth Green*
CHRISTOPHER PRIEST Inverted World*
BOLESŁAW PRUS The Doll*
RAYMOND QUENEAU We Always Treat Women Too Well
RAYMOND QUENEAU Witch Grass
RAYMOND RADIGUET Count d'Orgel's Ball
FRIEDRICH RECK Diary of a Man in Despair*
JULES RENARD Nature Stories*
JEAN RENOIR Renoir, My Father
GREGOR VON REZZORI An Ermine in Czernopol*
GREGOR VON REZZORI Memoirs of an Anti-Semite*
GREGOR VON REZZORI The Snows of Yesteryear: Portraits for an Autobiography*
TIM ROBINSON Stones of Aran: Labyrinth
TIM ROBINSON Stones of Aran: Pilgrimage
MILTON ROKEACH The Three Christs of Ypsilanti*
FR. ROLFE Hadrian the Seventh
GILLIAN ROSE Love's Work
WILLIAM ROUGHEAD Classic Crimes
CONSTANCE ROURKE American Humor: A Study of the National Character
SAKI The Unrest-Cure and Other Stories; illustrated by Edward Gorey
TAYEB SALIH Season of Migration to the North
TAYEB SALIH The Wedding of Zein*
JEAN-PAUL SARTRE We Have Only This Life to Live: Selected Essays. 1939–1975
GERSHOM SCHOLEM Walter Benjamin: The Story of a Friendship*
DANIEL PAUL SCHREBER Memoirs of My Nervous Illness
JAMES SCHUYLER Alfred and Guinevere
JAMES SCHUYLER What's for Dinner?*
SIMONE SCHWARZ-BART The Bridge of Beyond*
LEONARDO SCIASCIA The Day of the Owl
LEONARDO SCIASCIA Equal Danger
LEONARDO SCIASCIA The Moro Affair
LEONARDO SCIASCIA To Each His Own
LEONARDO SCIASCIA The Wine-Dark Sea
VICTOR SEGALEN René Leys*
ANNA SEGHERS Transit*